Skin and Psyche

Edited By

Klas Nordlind

Department of Dermatology

Karolinska University Hospital

Solna, Stockholm

Sweden

&

Anna Zalewska-Janowska

Psychodermatology Department

Medical University of Lodz

Poland

Skin and Psyche

Editors: Klas Nordlind & Anna Zalewska-Janowska

(ISBN) eBook : 978-1-68108-301-8

(ISBN) Print: 978-1-68108-302-5

First published in 2016.

Acknowledgement:

Declared none.

advertisements or ideas contained in the Work.

Limitation of Liability:

In no event will Bentham Science Publishers, its staff, editors and/or authors, be liable for any damages, including, without limitation, special, incidental and/or consequential damages and/or damages for lost data and/or profits arising out of (whether directly or indirectly) the use or inability to use the Work. The entire liability of Bentham Science Publishers shall be limited to the amount actually paid by you for the Work.

General:

1. Any dispute or claim arising out of or in connection with this License Agreement or the Work (including non-contractual disputes or claims) will be governed by and construed in accordance with the laws of the U.A.E. as applied in the Emirate of Dubai. Each party agrees that the courts of the Emirate of Dubai shall have exclusive jurisdiction to settle any dispute or claim arising out of or in connection with this License Agreement or the Work (including non-contractual disputes or claims).
2. Your rights under this License Agreement will automatically terminate without notice and without the need for a court order if at any point you breach any terms of this License Agreement. In no event will any delay or failure by Bentham Science Publishers in enforcing your compliance with this License Agreement constitute a waiver of any of its rights.
3. You acknowledge that you have read this License Agreement, and agree to be bound by its terms and conditions. To the extent that any other terms and conditions presented on any website of Bentham Science Publishers conflict with, or are inconsistent with, the terms and conditions set out in this License Agreement, you acknowledge that the terms and conditions set out in this License Agreement shall prevail.

Bentham Science Publishers Ltd.
Executive Suite Y - 2
PO Box 7917, Saif Zone
Sharjah, U.A.E.
Email: subscriptions@benthamscience.org

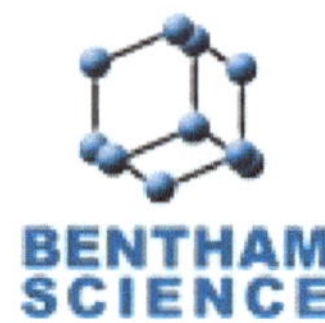

CONTENTS

FOREWORD

Psychodermatology is a critically important aspect of dermatological practice because psychological factors significantly affect a large proportion of our patients. It is an entire field, not just one disease, such as psoriasis. As such, there are different areas within psychodermatology. One important area is psychophysiological disorders, whereby emotional stress frequently precipitates or exacerbates real skin condition. This is most often observed in inflammatory conditions, such as psoriasis and eczema, but the influence of stress is also often reported in conditions without observable inflammation, such as vitiligo and alopecia areata. Another important area involves primary psychiatric disorder in which there are no real skin disorders; the lesions are all self-induced. This area includes delusion of parasitosis, neurotic excoriations, trichotillomania, and factitious dermatitis. The third important area is secondary psychiatric disorder where patient suffers from the negative consequence of disfigurement, such as depression, anxiety, and social phobia. Lastly, psychodermatology includes cutaneous sensory disorder where patient experiences distressing symptoms without visible primary skin lesions or diagnosable internal condition.

This book on psychodermatology covers different areas. Moreover, within these areas, there are highly relevant diagnoses such as, skin picking and body dysmorphic disorder, which are discussed in detail in separate chapters. I highly recommend any practitioners of dermatology to familiarize himself/herself with psychodermatology through this clinically useful book that is easily accessible. The material in this book will undoubtedly greatly enhance our care of these patients who are the most unfortunate and miserable sufferers of psychodermatological disorders.

John Koo
Argentina Leon
UCSF Department of Dermatology
San Francisco
California
USA

PREFACE

Psychodermatology is a part of general dermatology. As dermatologists, we will definitely meet patients with parasite delusions and, neurotic excoriation/artefacts, dysmorphofobia, or stress-worsened eczema.

This area meets several challenges, such as economy and difficulties to assess the outcomes for the patients. At the same time, the area of psychodermatology has a substantial developmental capacity. This goes for patient's clinical treatment as well as for more theoretical research.

Anna Zalewska-Janowska and I first met at an European Society of Dermatovenerology (EADV) conference in Gothenburg, and we decided to, together with experts in the respective fields, form this e-book in order to shed light on this important part of dermatology. Subsequently, we organized a few sessions on the Neurobiology of the Skin at European Society for Dermatological Research (ESDR) Congresses.

This e-book mainly aims at creating an interest for psychodermatology in dermatologists, both hospital based and colleagues working as private practitioners. Important issues dealing with chronic inflammatory diseases, facial dermatoses, artefacts, dysmorphophobia, parasite delusions, and therapeutic steps are dealt with.

Klas Nordlind
Department of Dermatology
Karolinska University Hospital, Solna
Stockholm
Sweden
&
Anna Zalewska-Janowska
Psychodermatology Department
Medical University of Lodz
Poland

List of Contributors

A. Bewley	Departments of Dermatology, Whipps Cross University Hospital, and The Royal London Hospital, London, UK
C. Bundy	The Dermatology Research Centre and Manchester Centre for Health Psychology, The University of Manchester, Manchester Academic Health Science Centre, Manchester, UK
AWM Ewers	Medical and Neuropsychology Unit, Faculty of Social and Behavioral Science, Leiden University, Institute of Psychology, Health, Leiden, Department of Medical Psychology, Radboud University Medical Centre, Nijmegen, The Netherlands
S. Friberg	Psykiatri Nordväst, Karolinska University Hospital, Solna, Sweden
V. Leibovici	Department of Dermatology, Hadassah-Hebrew University Medical Center, Jerusalem, Israel
S.B. Lonne-Rahm	Department of Dermatology, Mälarsjukhuset, Eskilstuna, and Dermatology and Venereology Unit, Department of Medicine, Solna, Karolinska Institutet, Stockholm, Sweden
M. Malakouti	Palo Alto Foundation Medical Group, Department of Dermatology, Mountain View, CA, USA
S.E. Marron	Alcañiz Hospital, University of Zaragoza, Aragon Health Sciences Institute (IACS), Zaragoza, Spain
S.R. McBride	Department of Dermatology, Royal Free NHS Foundation Trust, London, UK
A. Menter	Department of Dermatology, Baylor University Medical Center, Dallas, USA
L. Misery	Department of Dermatology, University Hospital of Brest, France
A. Mizara	Department of Dermatology, Royal Free NHS Foundation Trust, London, UK
P. Mohandas	Departments of Dermatology, Whipps Cross University Hospital, UK
K. Nordlind	Department of Dermatology, Karolinska University Hospital, Solna, Sweden
D. Radu-Djurfeldt	Psykiatri Sydväst, M46, Karolinska University Hospital, Huddinge, Sweden
Koulil S. Spillekom-van	Health, Medical and Neuropsychology Unit, Faculty of Social and Behavioral Science, Leiden University, Institute of Psychology, Leiden Department of Medical Psychology, Radboud University Medical Centre, Nijmegen, The Netherlands
L. Tomas Aragones	University of Zaragoza, Aragon Health Sciences Institute (IACS), Zaragoza, Spain

J.C. Ulnik	Pathophysiology and Psychosomatic diseases, Psychology School, Buenos Aires University, Buenos Aires, Argentina Argentine Psychoanalytical Association / Mental Health Department, Medicine School, Buenos Aires University, Buenos Aires, Argentina
S. Van Beugen	Institute of Psychology, Health, Medical and Neuropsychology Unit, Faculty of Social and Behavioral Science, Leiden University, Leiden, The Netherlands Department of Medical Psychology, Radboud University Medical Centre, Nijmegen, The Netherlands
A. Zalewska-Janowska	Medical University of Lodz, Psychodermatology Department, Poland

Skin and Psyche

2

CHAPTER 1

Skin and Psyche: Biological Aspects

Laurent Misery*

Department of Dermatology, University Hospital of Brest, 2 avenue Foch, 29200 Brest, France

Abstract: The skin has a dense innervation with synapses between nerve endings and many cells. These cells communicate *via* neurotransmitters and their receptors. Thus, the nervous system may influence different skin functions, including immunity. In skin diseases, the equilibrium of these neurotransmitters is disturbed. There are numerous disorders of this neuro-immuno-cutaneous system (NEICS). The present chapter aims at understanding the impact of psyche in inflammatory skin disorders.

Keywords: Itch, Nerve, Neurotransmitters, Pruritus, Psyche, Skin, Stress.

INTRODUCTION

Frequent interactions exist between the skin and the psyche. These interactions are understood through the organization of the neuro-immuno-cutaneous system (NEICS) [1, 2], and its interactions [3, 4].

INNERVATION OF THE SKIN

The skin is the organ of touch, this being necessary for human homeostasis. The absence of touch may be followed by death, such as reported in congenital pain insensitivity [5]. The skin is densely innervated, with nerve fibers up to its outermost layer [6]. This chapter aims to provide some data to illustrate that nerve endings are not only cellular endings in the skin in order to obtain information and transmit them to the central nervous system (CNS). But sensory and autonomic nerve endings are also involved in numerous interactions within the skin.

* **Corresponding author Laurent Misery:** Department of Dermatology, University Hospital of Brest, 2 avenue Foch, 29200 Brest, France; Tel: +3329822315; Fax: +33298223382; E-mail: laurent.misery@chu-best.fr.

Klas Nordlind & Anna Zalewska-Janowska (Eds.)

Anatomical Connections

Skin neurons have contacts with cutaneous cell endings, which contain neuro-secretory vesicles. These contacts may be viewed upon as synapses since the intercellular distance is less than 300 nm and being highly functional [7].

These contacts may be spontaneously produced *in vitro* (Fig. **1**).

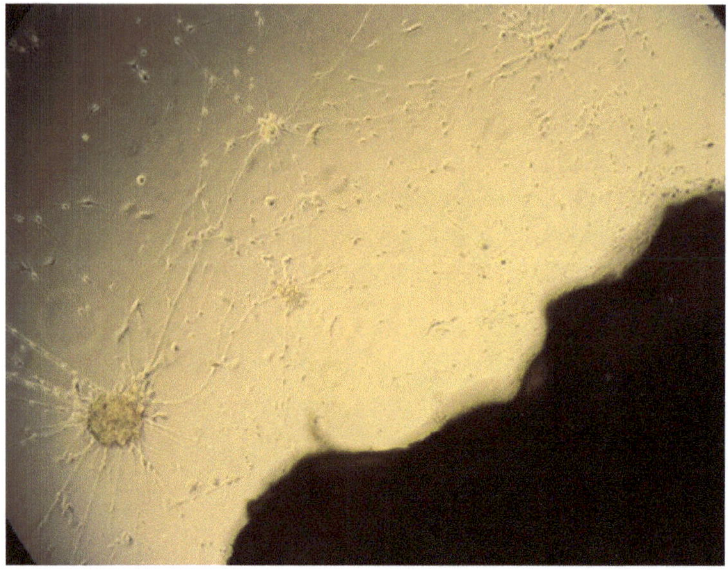

Fig. (1). *In vitro* co-culture of skin and neurons showing spontaneous growth of nerve endings from neurons (left) to the skin (right).

The first contacts between neurons and epidermal cells were described by Merkel [8], Merkel cells (or epidermal neuro-endocrine cells) being in contact with nerve endings [9]. Langerhans [10] also suspected the existence of such connections with Langerhans cells. These cells have then been shown to be in contact with axons *via* their cellular bodies [11, 12] and their dendrites [12]. In the epidermis, there are also contacts between nerve fibers and keratinocytes [13] and, more recently, connections with melanocytes have been reported [14].

In the dermis, there are contacts between nerve fibers and mast cells [15]. Recently dermal dendritic cells have been observed in contact with axons [16]. In contrast, perivascular nerves are found at the interface between the adventitia and the smooth muscle of the middle tunica layer [17].

Neurotransmitters

Among the numerous neurotransmitters (or neuromediators), about thirty are described in human skin (Table **1**) [18, 19]. Most are neuropeptides: bradykinin, calcitonin-gene related peptide (CGRP), gastrin-releasing peptide (GRP), neurokinins, neuropeptide Y (NPY), neurotensin, peptide histidine isoleucine (PHI), somatostatin (SOM), substance P, and vasoactive intestinal peptide (VIP). Others are neurohormones (adrenocorticotrophic hormone (ACTH), melanocyte-stimulating hormone (MSH), and prolactin), or catecholamines, endorphins, enkephalins, or acetylcholine (ACh). Nitric oxide (NO) is a more primitive, ancient skin neurotransmitter [20].

Table 1. Neurotransmitters in the skin.

Neuropeptides/neurohormones	Others
ACTH	ACh
CGRP	Angiotensin
CRH (corticotropin-releasing hormone)	DOPA
Endorphins	Dopamine
Enkephalins	Epinephrine
Galanin	Histamine
GRP	Norepinephrine
MSH	NO
Neurokinin A (NKA)	Serotonin
Neurokinin B (NKB)	
Neurotensin	
NPY	
PHI	
PHM (peptide histidine methionine)	
Prolactin	
PTH (parathyroid hormone)	
SOM	
Substance P	
VIP	

The quantity of skin neuromediators varies according to the individual, the disease, and their location. Neuropeptide concentrations range from 0.1 to 5.5 pmol/g of tissue [19].

Skin neuromediators are synthesized by nerve endings and Merkel cells but also by keratinocytes, Langerhans cells, melanocytes and immune cells (granulocytes, lymphocytes, monocytes-macrophages and especially mast cells). Neuro-secretory granules have been described only in nerve endings and Merkel cells, the mechanisms of neurotransmitter synthesis by other cells remaining unknown. The majority of the cutaneous cells have also been shown to possess receptors for the neuromediators [1].

Skin Cells Have Neuronal Capacities

Hence, like nerve cells, skin cells are able to express neuronal markers, receptors for neurotransmitters and produce neuromediators [4].

An epithelial or a neural origin of Merkel cells has been a matter of controversy [21 - 23]. However, it is now admitted that Merkel cells originate from epidermal stem cells [24]. These cells have certain nerve cell characteristics ((protein S-100, specific neuronal enolase, neurofilament protein, protein gene product (PGP) 9.5, chromogranin, synaptophysin)) and also show epithelial markers [22, 23]. They, furthermore, produce nerve growth factor (NGF) and its receptor. Merkel cells possess electric properties [25] and are mechanoreceptors [26]. They, as stated above, possess granules and neuro-secretory vesicles, containing neuropeptides. These granules are present in the entire cytoplasm, being more dense in juxta-axonal position [27].

They express chromogranin and their contents are intended for nerve and dermal cells, while the vesicles expressing synaptophysin, are located on the epidermal cell side [28]. Thus, human Merkel cells probably synthesize neuromediators, which are secreted by fusing granules in neurosecretory vesicles with the plasmic membrane. Through these neurotransmitters Merkel cells are able to modulate skin inflammation [29].

Langerhans cells and their precursors express proteins usually encountered in cells of the nervous system, *i.e.* protein S-100 and specific neuronal enolase [30, 31]. When being denervated Langerhans cells are able to express PGP 9.5 [32, 33]. These cells produce pro-opiomelanocortin (precursor to ACTH, endorphins and MSH) [34]. Through receptors on the cell surface surface, neuromediators, CGRP [11], substance P [35], GRP [36] and α-MSH [37], may modulate Langerhans cell functions. Thus, Langerhans cells are linking skin, immunity and nervous system [38].

Keratinocytes are able to produce neuromediators: pro-opiomelanocortin [34], ACh [39] dopamine, epinephrine and norepinephrine [40], and substance P [41]. These cells express receptors to substance P [42 - 46], VIP [47], CGRP [47], NPY [47], GRP [36], ACh (muscarinic or nicotinic) [48, 49] and MSH [50].

Melanocytes express protein S-100 and enzymes involved in catecholamine synthesis [51]. These cells express MSH receptors and possibly also to melatonin [52]. Catecholamines may induce the expression of $\alpha 1$ adreno-receptors [53].

In the dermis, fibroblasts have receptors to bombesin, SOM and substance P [54], while in the hypodermis catecholamine receptors of type $\beta 1$, $\beta 2$ and $\beta 3$ are present on adipocytes [55].

FUNCTIONAL LINKS BETWEEN SKIN AND THE NERVOUS SYSTEM

An interdependence has been described between Merkel cells and cutaneous nerves [56], even though being facultative [57]. Merkel cells might offer metabolic support for axons. Eliminating the Merkel cells causes a higher excitability threshold for the nerve ending [58]. In addition, these cells might be regulating the nerve ending positions.

Neuromediators have effects on eccrine or apocrine glandular cells, endothelial cells, epidermal cells, fibroblasts, immune cells and muscle cells, most often *via* protein G coupled receptors.

Hence, substance P may inhibit antigen presentation, through NK-1-type receptors on both Langerhans cells and T lymphocytes [35]. In a similar murine model, CGRP inhibits antigen presentation [11]. Furthermore, such an incubation inhibits the induction of B7-2 in mice [59] and seems to limit the interleukin (IL)-1 and

IL-12 production by Langerhans cells and to augment the production of IL-10 [60]. The inhibitory effects of CGRP have also been reported *in vivo*. Thus, CGRP inhibits delayed hypersensitivity reactions *via* local action [61], which also seems in part responsible for the immunosuppression obtained by exposure to ultraviolet (UV) radiation [3].

Epinephrine reduces the proliferation of keratinocytes [62]. Catecholamines appear to be synthesized essentially by undifferentiated keratinocytes, as well as be able to induce the expression of β2 receptors, the stimulation of which seems to induce keratinocyte differentiation, while simultaneously decreasing the biosynthesis of catecholamines [63]. ACh alters both the adhesion and migration of keratinocytes, cultured *in vitro,* through its nicotinic receptor [64, 65].

Substance P has variable effects on keratinocyte proliferation, *i.e.* stimulation [66, 67] or inhibition of the induction of VIP on proliferation [68]. Moreover, substance P increases the synthesis of cytokines IL-1α and β, IL-1 receptor antagonist, tumour necrosis factor (TNF)-α, IL-8, and also the expression of intercellular adhesion molecule (ICAM)-1 [69]. Bradykinin promotes the proto-oncogenes c-*fos,* c-*jun* and c-*myc* in keratinocytes [70].

Hence, neuromediators are able to modulate functions of all cellular types of the skin [71 - 76].

The Neuro-immuno-cutaneous System

Neuro-endocrine, immune systems and skin share properties and relationships allowing a common function. We have proposed the concept of the NEICS [77], these three systems being closely linked. There are physical linkages, contacts between nerve fibers, cutaneous and immune cells; and chemical linkages, cutaneous secretion of neuromediators and cell receptors for these. There are also functional linkages, such as modulation of cutaneous and/or immune functions by these neuromediators, and interactions between nervous, immune system and skin during the course of skin disorders. All cells of NEICS communicate using a common language, the words of which, *i.e.* cytokines and neurotransmitters, mediate the maintenance of a cellular homeostasis.

Other chemical actors of the NEICS are neurotrophins: NGF, brain-derived nerve factor (BDNF), neurotrophins 3 and 4 (NT-3 and NT-4). The neurotrophins are growth factors for neurons but also keratinocytes [78, 79]. They have anti-apoptotic effects, are involved in the release of neurotransmitters, control of inflammation [80], and hair growth and morphogenesis [81].

Such an organization is not skin specific. Thus, a NEICS analogue is also described in the gastro-intestinal (GI) tractus [82]. Contacts exist between nerve fibers and muscle cells, glandular cells, mast cells or lymphocytes. The nerve endings, but also lymphocytes, plasma cells and neuro-endocrine cells, secrete neuromediators. GI tractus cells, neuro-endocrine, muscle and glandular (or immune) cells possess receptors for neuromediators. In addition, neuromediators play a significant role in numerous symptoms/disorders of the GI tractus, *i.e.* inflammatory bowel disorders, *etc.*

WHEN THERE IS A SKIN DISORDER....

The nervous system plays a significant role in many skin disorders, especially inflammatory and/or auto-immune ones, *e.g.* psoriasis [83 - 88], atopic dermatitis [89 - 94], prurigo [95, 96], and vitiligo [97 - 99].

Psoriasis is a good example. One of its pathophysiological mechanisms is suggested to be psychological. Stress preceding psoriasis symptoms has been reported in varying degrees (from 32% to 90% of all cases) [83], and this by less than one month, and in two thirds of cases, less than two weeks. In addition, patients with psoriasis were reported to be more stress sensitive compared with a control group. In addition, the beneficial effects of psychotherapy or psychotropic drugs for psoriasis have been suggested. A psychiatric distress is presumably found in at least two-thirds of psoriasis patients [83]. However, psoriasis so far does not seem to occur due to a particular personality trait or a specific psychiatric disorder.

Psoriasis lesions often regress after surgical or traumatic denervation [84]. During the course of psoriasis, innervation increases, involving mainly intra-epidermal substance P- nerve fibers [100]. The affinity, distribution and amount of epidermal receptors to substance P are strongly modified [42]. Moreover, NGF levels increase in psoriatic skin [88]. In addition, blood levels of neuromediators, such as b-endorphin [86] are altered during flare-ups of psoriasis.

Atopic dermatitis is another good example of the effects of neuro-cutaneous alterations in skin disorders [94]. SP+ CGRP+ nerve fiber density increases, while adrenergic innervation decreases [89] and SOM-immunoreactive (IR) fibers disappear [90]. Distribution of epidermal and dermal SOM+cells is highly disrupted [91], whereas NPY-IR dendritic cells appear in the epidermis [101]. The concentration of substance P decreases while the level of VIP increases [92]. Prolactin blood levels are enhanced during atopic dermatitis outbreaks [93].

During the course of prurigo nodularis, the nerve fiber density increases and there is an excessive release of substance P, CGRP and VIP [95]. These neuropeptide modifications do not seem to be secondary to mechanical trauma from scratching, since not being found in lichenified skin.

During the course of vitiligo, the Koebner phenomenon is important [98]. Nerve fibers are damaged, showing both deterioration and regeneration [99]. The nerve fiber NPY immunoreactivity increases [99]. Contacts are observed between melanocytes and axons [102] and the synthesis of catecholamines by keratinocytes and melanocytes is impaired.

Thus, the list of skin diseases being possibly modulated by the activation of nerve endings is not limited. The nervous system is also important in the control of the effects of UV light in the skin [3], wound healing [103] as well as in cosmetic disorders [104], and sensitive skin [105].

SKIN AND STRESS

The course of many skin disorders may be influenced by psychological factors and stress events [106 - 108]. The links between psyche and skin appear to be intimate, especially when inflammation being substantially involved.

There are some psychogenic concepts to explain why the onset of cutaneous lesions can be triggered by psychological factors and/or life stress events [109 - 111]. Probably chemical factors, neurotransmitters and hormones, mediate an emotion or a stress into a cutaneous lesion [2].

Alterations of the NEICS are frequently observed in the course of numerous skin disorders. The levels of neuromediators are altered as well as the expression of their receptors or enzymes.

During a stress episode, similar phenomena occur in the nervous system and in the blood [112 - 117]. Thus, the skin production of mediators, such as substance P, is modified in response to stress [118]. Stress triggers mast cell degranulation through effects of local substance P and neurotensin [119]. In addition, dendritic cell functions are impaired by psychological stress *via* the release of substance P [120]. Serotonin [121] is another neurotransmitter with a potential role in such interactions.

However, stress does not induce psoriasis or other dermatoses in all patients. Firstly, the occurrence of a cutaneous disorder after stress appears to be linked to particular personality profiles and maybe to altered neurotransmitter profiles in response to stress. As a second option, this occurrence is linked to genetic and immune backgrounds.

Stress induces both local tissue releases of neurotransmitters and blood release of cortisol and catecholamines [122]. The response by the hypothalamic-pituitar--adrenal (HPA) axis is important in this respect [123]. This axis is characterized by a hierarchy in which the hypothalamus produces CRH, which induces the release of ACTH by the pituitary gland, in turn inducing the release of cortisol by adrenocortical glands [124]. Interestingly human skin itself also expresses molecules of the HPA axis, including pro-opiomelanocortin, CRH, the CRH receptor-1 (CRH-R1), and key enzymes related to corticosteroid synthesis. Also skin cells are able to synthesize glucocorticoids. Expression of these elements is organized into functional, cell type-specific regulatory loops, imitating the HPA axis, where differential CRH-driven responses of defined cutaneous cell populations are activated during stress.

ITCH

Itch (or pruritus) has been defined as an unpleasant sensation leading to the need of scratching [125]. The sensation of itch emanates from nerve fibres especially in the dermo-epidermal junction area [126]. In contrast inflammation of the reticular dermis or the hypodermis causes pain. Pruritic inflammatory dermatoses involving the epidermis and the superficial dermis have been reported to be associated with a higher number of free nerve endings [127].

The identification of specific or selective itch receptors– pruriceptors–in the skin, has been a major discovery. In microneurography experiments C fibres, unresponsive to mechanical or heat stimulation, but being activated by iontophoresis of histamine, have been identified [128]. Since these fibres could be weakly activated by capsaicin and certain other substances, they were termed 'itch-selective', rather than 'itch-specific' [129]. Nociceptors and pruriceptors are usually localized on the same nerve endings [130]. This overlap may explain why neuropathic itch is rarely the sole symptom.

In addition a histamine-independent pathway–initially found to be activated by cowhage spicules–has been reported [131]. This subset of nerve endings has been shown to be activated by cysteine or serine proteases, including mucunain (a protease from cowhage) *via* the proteinase-activated receptor (PAR)-2 or PAR-4 [132].

In addition an Aδ, itch-specific subset of both histamine- and capsaicin-sensitive nerve fibres, and possibly being different from skin flare mediating fibres, has been described [133].

However, many other mediators, especially neurotransmitters [134] have been reported to affect itch without selective action on a specific nerve ending subset. Other specific pathways might further on be identified.

In the spinal cord, there is a specific neuron subset being involved in itch [135]. Also in the brain subsets of cowhage-sensitive and histamine-responsive neurons, are found, being involved in pruritus perception [134]. In the thalamus, both sets of neurons have axons terminating in the contralateral ventral posterior lateral, ventral posterior inferior, and posterior nuclei. Cowhage neurons have additional projections to the contralateral suprageniculate and medial geniculate nuclei [136]. After these initial findings [137], functional neuroimaging studies have indicated cortical and subcortical regions implicated in itch [138]. Moreover, the neuronal networks processing the two types of itch are partially overlapping

[139].

The 'itch centers' in the brain may allow us to understand how itch can be modulated, and sometimes initiated locally, and how stress and other psychological factors are able to modulate its perception. This relationship between itch and stress has been especially studied in atopic dermatitis patients [140]. Such patients often report a close relationship between emotional distress, pruritus, and scratching [140, 141].

CONCLUSION

All these discoveries may increase our understanding of the interactions between skin and the psyche in skin disorders, being aggravated by psychological factors (Table **2**).

Table 2. Classification of psychocutaneous disorders [from ref.142].

1. Psychological disorders secondary to skin disorders
2. Psychological disorders responsible for skin disorders
2.1. Psychological disorders responsible for psychogenic skin sensations
2.1.1.Delusional syndromes (*e.g.* delusional parasitosis, hypochondria)
2.1.2. Phobias (*e.g.* dysmorphophobia, bromidrosophobia)
2.1.3. Psychogenic pruritus
2.1.4. Psychogenic dysesthesia and paresthesia
2.1.5. Pain syndromes (*e.g.* glossodynia, vulvodynia, anodynia)
2.2. Psychological disorders responsible for skin lesions
2.2.1. Severe (*e.g.* dermatitis artefacta, psychogenic excoriations)
2.2.2. Not severe (*e.g.* trichotillomania)
3. Skin disorders influenced by mental disorders
3.1. Dermatological diseases (*e.g.* atopic dermatitis, psoriasis, urticaria)
3.2. Cosmetological disorders (*e.g.* telogen effluvium, skin aging)
4. Skin and mental disorders without any obvious relationship

CONFLICT OF INTEREST

The author is medical advisor to Almirall, Astellas, BASF, Bioderma, Clarins,

Galderma, GSK, Johnson & Johnson, Maruho, Novartis, Pierre Fabre, Solabia, and Uriage.

Part of this chapter has been previously published in G Ital Dermatol Venereol 2005;140:677-84.

ACKNOWLEDGEMENTS

Declared none.

REFERENCES

[1] Misery L. Skin, immunity and the nervous system. Br J Dermatol 1997; 137(6): 843-50. [http://dx.doi.org/10.1111/j.1365-2133.1997.tb01542.x] [PMID: 9470898]

[2] Misery L. Are biochemical mediators the missing link between psychosomatics and dermatology? Dermatol Psychosom 2001; 2: 178-83. [http://dx.doi.org/10.1159/000049668]

[3] Misery L. The neuro-immuno-cutaneous system and ultraviolet radiation. Photodermatol Photoimmunol Photomed 2000; 16(2): 78-81. [http://dx.doi.org/10.1034/j.1600-0781.2000.d01-8.x] [PMID: 10823317]

[4] Misery L. The interactions between skin and nervous system. G Ital Dermatol Venereol 2005; 140: 677-84.

[5] Misery L, Hermier M, Staniek V, *et al.* Congenital insensitivity to pain with anhidrosis: absence of substance P receptors in the skin. Br J Dermatol 1999; 140(1): 190-1. [http://dx.doi.org/10.1046/j.1365-2133.1999.02694.x] [PMID: 10215808]

[6] Wang L, Hilliges M, Jernberg T, Wiegleb-Edström D, Johansson O. Protein gene product 9.5-immunoreactive nerve fibres and cells in human skin. Cell Tissue Res 1990; 261(1): 25-33. [http://dx.doi.org/10.1007/BF00329435] [PMID: 2143435]

[7] Chateau Y, Misery L. Connections between nerve endings and epidermal cells: are they synapses? Exp Dermatol 2004; 13(1): 2-4. [http://dx.doi.org/10.1111/j.0906-6705.2004.00158.x] [PMID: 15009109]

[8] Merkel F. Tastzellen und Tastkorperchen bei den Haustieren und beim Menschen. Arch Mikrosk Anat 1875; 11: 636-52. [http://dx.doi.org/10.1007/BF02933819]

[9] Hartschuh W, Weihe E. Fine structural analysis of the synaptic junction of Merkel cell-axo--complexes. J Invest Dermatol 1980; 75(2): 159-65. [http://dx.doi.org/10.1111/1523-1747.ep12522555] [PMID: 6774030]

[10] Langerhans P. Uber die Nerven der menschlichen Haut. Virchows Arch Pathol Anat Physiol 1868; 44: 325-37. [http://dx.doi.org/10.1007/BF01959006]

[11] Hosoi J, Murphy GF, Egan CL, *et al.* Regulation of Langerhans cell function by nerves containing calcitonin gene-related peptide. Nature 1993; 363(6425): 159-63. [http://dx.doi.org/10.1038/363159a0] [PMID: 8483499]

[12] Gaudillere A, Misery L, Souchier C, Claudy A, Schmitt D. Intimate associations between PGP9.5-positive nerve fibres and Langerhans cells. Br J Dermatol 1996; 135(2): 343-4. [http://dx.doi.org/10.1111/j.1365-2133.1996.tb01191.x] [PMID: 8881702]

[13] Hilliges M, Wang L, Johansson O. Ultrastructural evidence for nerve fibers within all vital layers of the human epidermis. J Invest Dermatol 1995; 104(1): 134-7. [http://dx.doi.org/10.1111/1523-1747.ep12613631] [PMID: 7798631]

[14] Hara M, Toyoda M, Yaar M, *et al.* Innervation of melanocytes in human skin. J Exp Med 1996; 184(4): 1385-95. [http://dx.doi.org/10.1084/jem.184.4.1385] [PMID: 8879211]

[15] Wiesner-Menzel L, Schulz B, Vakilzadeh F, Czarnetzki BM. Electron microscopical evidence for a direct contact between nerve fibres and mast cells. Acta Derm Venereol 1981; 61(6): 465-9. [PMID: 6177155]

[16] Sueki H, Telegan B, Murphy GF. Computer-assisted three-dimensional reconstruction of human dermal dendrocytes. J Invest Dermatol 1995; 105(5): 704-8. [http://dx.doi.org/10.1111/1523-1747.ep12324502] [PMID: 7594648]

[17] Chédotal A, Hamel E. L'innervation cholinergique de la paroi vasculaire. Med Sci (Paris) 1993; 9: 1035-42. [http://dx.doi.org/10.4267/10608/2806]

[18] Lotti T, Hautmann G, Panconesi E. Neuropeptides in skin. J Am Acad Dermatol 1995; 33(3): 482-96. [http://dx.doi.org/10.1016/0190-9622(95)91395-5] [PMID: 7657872]

[19] Eedy DJ, Shaw C, Johnston CF, Buchanan KD. The regional distribution of neuropeptides in human skin as assessed by radioimmunoassay and high-performance liquid chromatography. Clin Exp Dermatol 1994; 19(6): 463-72. [http://dx.doi.org/10.1111/j.1365-2230.1994.tb01248.x] [PMID: 7534221]

[20] Boissel JP, Ohly D, Bros M, Gödtel-Armbrust U, Förstermann U, Frank S. The neuronal nitric oxide synthase is upregulated in mouse skin repair and in response to epidermal growth factor in human HaCaT keratinocytes. J Invest Dermatol 2004; 123(1): 132-9. [http://dx.doi.org/10.1111/j.0022-202X.2004.22731.x] [PMID: 15191553]

[21] Boulais N, Misery L. Merkel cells. J Am Acad Dermatol 2007; 57(1): 147-65. [http://dx.doi.org/10.1016/j.jaad.2007.02.009] [PMID: 17412453]

[22] Gaudillère A, Misery L. [Merkel cell]. Ann Dermatol Venereol 1994; 121(12): 909-17. [PMID: 7632011]

[23] Moll I, Hartscuh W, Moll R. First International Merkel Symposium, Heidelberg, Germany. J Invest Dermatol 1995; 105: 851-3. [http://dx.doi.org/10.1111/1523-1747.ep12326653]

[24] Woo SH, Stumpfova M, Jensen UB, Lumpkin EA, Owens DM. Identification of epidermal progenitors for the Merkel cell lineage. Development 2010; 137(23): 3965-71.

[http://dx.doi.org/10.1242/dev.055970] [PMID: 21041368]

[25] Yamashita Y, Akaike N, Wakamori M, Ikeda I, Ogawa H. Voltage-dependent currents in isolated single Merkel cells of rats. J Physiol 1992; 450: 143-62.
[http://dx.doi.org/10.1113/jphysiol.1992.sp019120] [PMID: 1331421]

[26] Boulais N, Pennec JP, Lebonvallet N, *et al.* Rat Merkel cells are mechanoreceptors and osmoreceptors. PLoS One 2009; 4(11): e7759.
[http://dx.doi.org/10.1371/journal.pone.0007759] [PMID: 19898622]

[27] Hartschuh W, Weihe E. Multiple messenger candidates and marker substance in the mammalian Merkel cell-axon complex: a light and electron microscopic immunohistochemical study. Prog Brain Res 1988; 74: 181-7.
[http://dx.doi.org/10.1016/S0079-6123(08)63012-5] [PMID: 3187030]

[28] Ortonne JP, Petchot-Bacque JP, Verrando P, Pisani A, Pautrat G, Bernerd F. Normal Merkel cells express a synaptophysin-like immunoreactivity. Dermatologica 1988; 177(1): 1-10.
[http://dx.doi.org/10.1159/000248491] [PMID: 3141225]

[29] Boulais N, Pereira U, Lebonvallet N, *et al.* Merkel cells as putative regulatory cells in skin disorders: an *in vitro* study. PLoS One 2009; 4(8): e6528.
[http://dx.doi.org/10.1371/journal.pone.0006528] [PMID: 19668696]

[30] Cocchia D, Michetti F, Donato R. Immunochemical and immuno-cytochemical localization of S-100 antigen in normal human skin. Nature 1981; 294(5836): 85-7.
[http://dx.doi.org/10.1038/294085a0] [PMID: 7290214]

[31] Misery L, Campos L, Sabido O, *et al.* S100 protein and neuron-specific enolase on monocytic leukemic CD1+ cells, probable precursors of Langerhans cells. Eur J Haematol 1993; 51(3): 132-5.
[http://dx.doi.org/10.1111/j.1600-0609.1993.tb00612.x] [PMID: 7691652]

[32] Hsieh ST, Choi S, Lin WM, Chang YC, Mcarthur JC, Griffin JW. Epidermal denervation and its effects on keratinocytes and Langerhans cells. J Neurocytol 1996; 25(9): 513-24.
[http://dx.doi.org/10.1007/BF02284819] [PMID: 8910797]

[33] Hamzeh H, Gaudillère A, Sabido O, *et al.* Expression of PGP9.5 on Langerhans' cells and their precursors. Acta Derm Venereol 2000; 80(1): 14-6.
[http://dx.doi.org/10.1080/000155500750012423] [PMID: 10721824]

[34] Bhardwaj RS, Luger TA. Proopiomelanocortin production by epidermal cells: evidence for an immune neuroendocrine network in the epidermis. Arch Dermatol Res 1994; 287(1): 85-90.
[http://dx.doi.org/10.1007/BF00370724] [PMID: 7726641]

[35] Staniek V, Misery L, Péguet-Navarro J, *et al.* Binding and *in vitro* modulation of human epidermal Langerhans cell functions by substance P. Arch Dermatol Res 1997; 289(5): 285-91.
[http://dx.doi.org/10.1007/s004030050194] [PMID: 9164639]

[36] Staniek V, Misery L, Peguet-Navarro J, *et al.* Expression of gastrin-releasing peptide receptor in human skin. Acta Derm Venereol 1996; 76(4): 282-6.
[PMID: 8869685]

[37] Shimizu T, Streilein JW. Influence of alpha-melanocyte stimulating hormone on induction of contact hypersensitivity and tolerance. J Dermatol Sci 1994; 8(3): 187-93.

[http://dx.doi.org/10.1016/0923-1811(94)90053-1] [PMID: 7865476]

[38] Misery L. Langerhans cells in the neuro-immuno-cutaneous system. J Neuroimmunol 1998; 89(1-2): 83-7.
[http://dx.doi.org/10.1016/S0165-5728(98)00117-9] [PMID: 9726829]

[39] Grando SA, Kist DA, Qi M, Dahl MV. Human keratinocytes synthesize, secrete, and degrade acetylcholine. J Invest Dermatol 1993; 101(1): 32-6.
[http://dx.doi.org/10.1111/1523-1747.ep12358588] [PMID: 8331294]

[40] Schallreuter KU, Wood JM, Lemke R, *et al.* Production of catecholamines in the human epidermis. Biochem Biophys Res Commun 1992; 189(1): 72-8.
[http://dx.doi.org/10.1016/0006-291X(92)91527-W] [PMID: 1360208]

[41] Bae S, Matsunaga Y, Tanaka Y, Katayama I. Autocrine induction of substance P mRNA and peptide in cultured normal human keratinocytes. Biochem Biophys Res Commun 1999; 263(2): 327-33.
[http://dx.doi.org/10.1006/bbrc.1999.1285] [PMID: 10491292]

[42] Staniek V, Doutremepuich J, Schmitt D, Claudy A, Misery L. Expression of substance P receptors in normal and psoriatic skin. Pathobiology 1999; 67(1): 51-4.
[http://dx.doi.org/10.1159/000028051] [PMID: 9873229]

[43] Arenberger P, Leder RO, Abraham A, Chang JK, Farber EM. Substance P binding in normal neonatal foreskin. Br J Dermatol 1995; 132(1): 54-8.
[http://dx.doi.org/10.1111/j.1365-2133.1995.tb08624.x] [PMID: 7538777]

[44] Keményi L, von Restorff B, Michel G, Ruzicka T. Specific binding and lack of growth-promoting activity of substance P in cultured human keratinocytes. J Invest Dermatol 1994; 103(4): 605-6.
[http://dx.doi.org/10.1111/1523-1747.ep12396976] [PMID: 7523535]

[45] Pincelli C, Fantini F, Giardino L, *et al.* Autoradiographic detection of substance P receptors in normal and psoriatic skin. J Invest Dermatol 1993; 101(3): 301-4.
[http://dx.doi.org/10.1111/1523-1747.ep12365423] [PMID: 7690377]

[46] Song IS, Bunnett NW, Olerud JE, *et al.* Substance P induction of murine keratinocyte PAM 212 interleukin 1 production is mediated by the neurokinin 2 receptor (NK-2R). Exp Dermatol 2000; 9(1): 42-52.
[http://dx.doi.org/10.1034/j.1600-0625.2000.009001042.x] [PMID: 10688374]

[47] Takahashi K, Nakanishi S, Imamura S. Direct effects of cutaneous neuropeptides on adenylyl cyclase activity and proliferation in a keratinocyte cell line: stimulation of cyclic AMP formation by CGRP and VIP/PHM, and inhibition by NPY through G protein-coupled receptors. J Invest Dermatol 1993; 101(5): 646-51.
[http://dx.doi.org/10.1111/1523-1747.ep12371670] [PMID: 8228323]

[48] Grando SA, Horton RM, Pereira EF, *et al.* A nicotinic acetylcholine receptor regulating cell adhesion and motility is expressed in human keratinocytes. J Invest Dermatol 1995; 105(6): 774-81.
[http://dx.doi.org/10.1111/1523-1747.ep12325606] [PMID: 7490471]

[49] Grando SA, Zelickson BD, Kist DA, *et al.* Keratinocyte muscarinic acetylcholine receptors: immunolocalization and partial characterization. J Invest Dermatol 1995; 104(1): 95-100.
[http://dx.doi.org/10.1111/1523-1747.ep12613582] [PMID: 7528248]

[50] Chakraborty A, Slominski A, Ermak G, Hwang J, Pawelek J. Ultraviolet B and melanocyte-stimulating hormone (MSH) stimulate mRNA production for alpha MSH receptors and proopiomelanocortin-derived peptides in mouse melanoma cells and transformed keratinocytes. J Invest Dermatol 1995; 105(5): 655-9.
[http://dx.doi.org/10.1111/1523-1747.ep12324134] [PMID: 7594638]

[51] Schallreuter KU, Wood JM, Pittelkow MR, *et al.* Increased monoamine oxidase A activity in the epidermis of patients with vitiligo. Arch Dermatol Res 1996; 288(1): 14-8.
[http://dx.doi.org/10.1007/BF02505037] [PMID: 8750929]

[52] Almeida AL, Markus RP, Visconti MA, Castrucci AM. Presence of melatonin binding sites in S-91 murine melanoma cells. Pigment Cell Res 1995; 10: 31.

[53] Schallreuter KU, Körner C, Pittelkow MR, Swanson NN, Gardner ML. The induction of the alpha--adrenoceptor signal transduction system on human melanocytes. Exp Dermatol 1996; 5(1): 20-3.
[http://dx.doi.org/10.1111/j.1600-0625.1996.tb00088.x] [PMID: 8624607]

[54] Gaudillère A, Bernard C, Abello J, Schmitt D, Claudy A, Misery L. Human normal dermal fibroblasts express somatostatin receptors. Exp Dermatol 1999; 8(4): 267-73.
[http://dx.doi.org/10.1111/j.1600-0625.1999.tb00381.x] [PMID: 10439224]

[55] Arner P. The beta 3-adrenergic receptor--a cause and cure of obesity? N Engl J Med 1995; 333(6): 382-3.
[http://dx.doi.org/10.1056/NEJM199508103330612] [PMID: 7609759]

[56] Morohunfola KA, Jones TE, Munger BL. The differentiation of the skin and its appendages. I. Normal development of papillary ridges. Anat Rec 1992; 232(4): 587-98.
[http://dx.doi.org/10.1002/ar.1092320414] [PMID: 1554108]

[57] Narisawa Y, Kohda H. Merkel cells do not require trophic maintenance from the nerves in adult human skin. Br J Dermatol 1995; 133(4): 553-6.
[http://dx.doi.org/10.1111/j.1365-2133.1995.tb02703.x] [PMID: 7577582]

[58] Diamond J, Holmes M, Nurse CA. Are Merkel cell-neurite reciprocal synapses involved in the initiation of tactile responses in salamander skin? J Physiol 1986; 376: 101-20.
[http://dx.doi.org/10.1113/jphysiol.1986.sp016144] [PMID: 3795072]

[59] Gillardon F, Moll I, Michel S, Benrath J, Weihe E, Zimmerman M. CGRP and nitric oxide are involved in ultraviolet radiation-induced immunosuppression. Eur J Pharmacol 1995; 296: 395-400.
[http://dx.doi.org/10.1016/0926-6917(95)90060-8] [PMID: 8748693]

[60] Hosoi J, Torii H, Fox F, Zan Z, Rook AH, Granstein RD. Alteration of cytokine expression by calcitonin gene-related peptide (CGRP). J Invest Dermatol 1995; 105: 859.

[61] Asahina A, Hosoi J, Beissert S, Stratigos A, Granstein RD. Inhibition of the induction of delayed-type and contact hyeprsensitivity by CGRP. J Immunol 1995; 154: 3056-61.
[PMID: 7897198]

[62] Clausen OP, Thorud E, Iversen OH. Adrenalin has differential effects on epidermal cell cycle progression in mice. J Invest Dermatol 1982; 78(6): 472-6.
[http://dx.doi.org/10.1111/1523-1747.ep12510172] [PMID: 7086167]

[63] Schallreuter KU, Lemke KR, Pittelkow MR, Wood JM, Körner C, Malik R. Catecholamines in human keratinocyte differentiation. J Invest Dermatol 1995; 104(6): 953-7. [http://dx.doi.org/10.1111/1523-1747.ep12606218] [PMID: 7769265]

[64] Misery L. Nicotine effects on skin: are they positive or negative? Exp Dermatol 2004; 13(11): 665-70. [http://dx.doi.org/10.1111/j.0906-6705.2004.00274.x] [PMID: 15500638]

[65] Grando SA, Horton RM, Mauro TM, Kist DA, Lee TX, Dahl MV. Activation of keratinocyte nicotinic cholinergic receptors stimulates calcium influx and enhances cell differentiation. J Invest Dermatol 1996; 107(3): 412-8. [http://dx.doi.org/10.1111/1523-1747.ep12363399] [PMID: 8751979]

[66] Paus R, Heinzelmann T, Robicsek S, Czarnetzki BM, Maurer M. Substance P stimulates murine epidermal keratinocyte proliferation and dermal mast cell degranulation in situ. Arch Dermatol Res 1995; 287(5): 500-2. [http://dx.doi.org/10.1007/BF00373436] [PMID: 7542862]

[67] Tanaka T, Danno K. K. I, Imamura S. Effects of substance P and substance K on the growth of keratinocytes. J Invest Dermatol 1988; 90: 399-401. [http://dx.doi.org/10.1111/1523-1747.ep12456487] [PMID: 2450147]

[68] Pincelli C, Fantini F, Romualdi P, *et al.* Substance P is diminished and vasoactive intestinal peptide is augmented in psoriatic lesions and these peptides exert disparate effects on the proliferation of cultured human keratinocytes. J Invest Dermatol 1992; 98(4): 421-7. [http://dx.doi.org/10.1111/1523-1747.ep12499846] [PMID: 1372339]

[69] Viac J, Guéniche A, Doutremepuich JD, Reichert U, Claudy A, Schmitt D. Substance P and keratinocyte activation markers: an in vitro approach. Arch Dermatol Res 1996; 288(2): 85-90. [http://dx.doi.org/10.1007/BF02505049] [PMID: 8932586]

[70] Coutant KD, Ryder NS. Bradykinin upregulates immediate-early gene mRNA in human keratinocytes. Arch Dermatol Res 1996; 288(1): 2-6. [http://dx.doi.org/10.1007/BF02505034] [PMID: 8750926]

[71] Ansel JC, Kaynard AH, Armstrong CA, Olerud J, Bunnett N, Payan D. Skin-nervous system interactions. J Invest Dermatol 1996; 106(1): 198-204. [http://dx.doi.org/10.1111/1523-1747.ep12330326] [PMID: 8592075]

[72] Lambert RW, Granstein RD. Neuropeptides and Langerhans cells. Exp Dermatol 1998; 7(2-3): 73-80. [http://dx.doi.org/10.1111/j.1600-0625.1998.tb00306.x] [PMID: 9583746]

[73] Lotti T, Bianchi B, Panconesi E. Neuropeptides and skin disorders. The new frontiers of neuro-endocrine-cutaneous immunology. Int J Dermatol 1999; 38(9): 673-5. [http://dx.doi.org/10.1046/j.1365-4362.1999.00767.x] [PMID: 10517683]

[74] Pincelli C, Fantini F, Giannetti A. Neuropeptides and skin inflammation. Dermatology (Basel) 1993; 187(3): 153-8. [http://dx.doi.org/10.1159/000247232] [PMID: 7693068]

[75] Scholzen T, Armstrong CA, Bunnett NW, Luger TA, Olerud JE, Ansel JC. Neuropeptides in the skin: interactions between the neuroendocrine and the skin immune systems. Exp Dermatol 1998; 7(2-3): 81-96.

[http://dx.doi.org/10.1111/j.1600-0625.1998.tb00307.x] [PMID: 9583747]

[76] Luger TA, Lotti T. Neuropeptides: role in inflammatory skin diseases. J Eur Acad Dermatol Venereol 1998; 10(3): 207-11.
[http://dx.doi.org/10.1111/j.1468-3083.1998.tb00736.x] [PMID: 9643321]

[77] Misery L. Le système neuro-immuno-cutané (SNIC). Pathol Biol (Paris) 1996; 44(10): 867-74.
[PMID: 9157366]

[78] Marconi A, Terracina M, Fila C, *et al.* Expression and function of neurotrophins and their receptors in cultured human keratinocytes. J Invest Dermatol 2003; 121(6): 1515-21.
[http://dx.doi.org/10.1111/j.1523-1747.2003.12624.x] [PMID: 14675204]

[79] Pincelli C, Fantini F, Giannetti A. Nerve growth factor and the skin. Int J Dermatol 1994; 33(5): 308-12.
[http://dx.doi.org/10.1111/j.1365-4362.1994.tb01058.x] [PMID: 8039967]

[80] Freund V, Kassel O, Frossard N. Le facteur de croissance des nerfs: un nouveau médiateur de l'inflammation? Rev Fr Allergol Immunol Clin 2001; 41: 571-8.
[http://dx.doi.org/10.1016/S0335-7457(01)00072-7]

[81] Botchkareva NV, Botchkarev VA, Albers KM, Metz M, Paus R. Distinct roles for nerve growth factor and brain-derived neurotrophic factor in controlling the rate of hair follicle morphogenesis. J Invest Dermatol 2000; 114(2): 314-20.
[http://dx.doi.org/10.1046/j.1523-1747.2000.00864.x] [PMID: 10651992]

[82] Stead RH. Innervation of mucosal immune cells in the gastrointestinal tract. Reg Immunol 1992; 4(2): 91-9.
[PMID: 1354471]

[83] Mazzetti M, Mozzetta A, Soavi GC, *et al.* Psoriasis, stress and psychiatry: psychodynamic characteristics of stressors. Acta Derm Venereol Suppl (Stockh) 1994; 186: 62-4.
[PMID: 8073841]

[84] Pincelli C, Fantini F, Magnoni C, Giannetti A. Psoriasis and the nervous system. Acta Derm Venereol Suppl (Stockh) 1994; 186: 60-1.
[PMID: 8073840]

[85] Al'Abadie MS, Kent GG, Gawkrodger DJ. The relationship between stress and the onset and exacerbation of psoriasis and other skin conditions. Br J Dermatol 1994; 130(2): 199-203.
[http://dx.doi.org/10.1111/j.1365-2133.1994.tb02900.x] [PMID: 8123572]

[86] Glinski W, Brodecka H, Glinska-Ferenz M, Kowalski D. Increased concentration of beta-endorphin in sera of patients with psoriasis and other inflammatory dermatoses. Br J Dermatol 1994; 131(2): 260-4.
[http://dx.doi.org/10.1111/j.1365-2133.1994.tb08502.x] [PMID: 7917992]

[87] Goicoechea M, de Sequera P, Ochando A, Andrea C, Caramelo C. Uremic pruritus: an unresolved problem in hemodialysis patients. Nephron 1999; 82(1): 73-4.
[http://dx.doi.org/10.1159/000045371] [PMID: 10224488]

[88] Fantini F, Magnoni C, Bracci-Laudiero L, Pincelli C TE. Nerve growth factor is increased in psoriatic skin. J Invest Dermatol 1995; 105(6): 854-5.
[http://dx.doi.org/10.1111/1523-1747.ep12326689] [PMID: 7490482]

[89] Cooper KD. Atopic dermatitis: recent trends in pathogenesis and therapy. J Invest Dermatol 1994; 102(1): 128-37.
[http://dx.doi.org/10.1111/1523-1747.ep12371746] [PMID: 8288906]

[90] Tobin D, Nabarro G, Baart de la Faille H, van Vloten WA, van der Putte SC, Schuurman HJ. Increased number of immunoreactive nerve fibers in atopic dermatitis. J Allergy Clin Immunol 1992; 90(4 Pt 1): 613-22.
[http://dx.doi.org/10.1016/0091-6749(92)90134-N] [PMID: 1383306]

[91] Pincelli C, Fantini F, Massimi P, Girolomoni G, Seidenari S, Giannetti A. Neuropeptides in skin from patients with atopic dermatitis: an immunohistochemical study. Br J Dermatol 1990; 122(6): 745-50.
[http://dx.doi.org/10.1111/j.1365-2133.1990.tb06261.x] [PMID: 1695105]

[92] Giannetti A, Fantini F, Cimitan A, Pincelli C. Vasoactive intestinal polypeptide and substance P in the pathogenesis of atopic dermatitis. Acta Derm Venereol Suppl (Stockh) 1992; 176: 90-2.
[PMID: 1282289]

[93] Rupprecht M, Renders U, Koch HU, Hornstein OP. Twenty-four hour secretion of prolactin in patients with atopic eczema and normal controls. Eur J Dermatol 1993; 3: 495-8.

[94] Misery L. Atopic dermatitis and the nervous system. Clin Rev Allergy Immunol 2011; 41(3): 259-66.
[http://dx.doi.org/10.1007/s12016-010-8225-z] [PMID: 21181506]

[95] Abadía Molina F, Burrows NP, Jones RR, Terenghi G, Polak JM. Increased sensory neuropeptides in nodular prurigo: a quantitative immunohistochemical analysis. Br J Dermatol 1992; 127(4): 344-51.
[http://dx.doi.org/10.1111/j.1365-2133.1992.tb00452.x] [PMID: 1419754]

[96] Al'Abadie MS, Senior HJ, Bleehen SS, Gawkrodger DJ. Neuronal marker and neuropeptide studies in nodular prurigo. Eur J Dermatol 1994; 4: 154-8.

[97] Morohashi M, Hashimoto K, Goodman TF Jr, Newton DE, Rist T. Ultrastructural studies of vitiligo, Vogt-Koyanagi syndrome, and incontinentia pigmenti achromians. Arch Dermatol 1977; 113(6): 755-66.
[http://dx.doi.org/10.1001/archderm.1977.01640060051004] [PMID: 869545]

[98] Gauthier Y. The importance of Koebner's phenomenon in the induction of vitiligo vulgaris lesions. Eur J Dermatol 1995; 5: 704-8.

[99] Al'Abadie MS, Warren MA, Bleehen SS, Gawkrodger DJ. Morphologic observations on the dermal nerves in vitiligo: an ultrastructural study. Int J Dermatol 1995; 34(12): 837-40.
[http://dx.doi.org/10.1111/j.1365-4362.1995.tb04417.x] [PMID: 8647660]

[100] Al'Abadie MS, Senior HJ, Bleehen SS, Gawkrodger DJ. Neuropeptides and general neuronal marker in psoriasis--an immunohistochemical study. Clin Exp Dermatol 1995; 20(5): 384-9.
[http://dx.doi.org/10.1111/j.1365-2230.1995.tb01354.x] [PMID: 8593714]

[101] Pincelli C, Fantini F. P. M, Gianetti A. Neuropeptide Y-like immunoreactivity in Langerhans cells from patients with atopic dermatitis. J Neurosci 1990; 51: 219-20.

[102] Al'Abadie MS, Senior HJ, Bleehen SS, Gawkrodger DJ. Neuropeptide and neuronal marker studies in vitiligo. Br J Dermatol 1994; 131(2): 160-5.
[http://dx.doi.org/10.1111/j.1365-2133.1994.tb08486.x] [PMID: 7522512]

[103] Chéret J, Lebonvallet N, Buhé V, Misery L, Le Gall-Ianotto C. Influence of neurotransmitters and NGF on human cutaneous wound healing process. Wound Repair Regen 2013; 21: 772-88. [PMID: 24134750]

[104] Misery L. Les nerfs à fleur de peau. Int J Cosmet Sci 2002; 24(2): 111-6. [http://dx.doi.org/10.1046/j.1467-2494.2002.00134.x] [PMID: 18498503]

[105] Misery L. Sensitive skin. Expert Rev Dermatol 2013; 8: 631-7. [http://dx.doi.org/10.1586/17469872.2013.856688]

[106] Panconesi E, Hautmann G. Psychophysiology of stress in dermatology. The psychobiologic pattern of psychosomatics. Dermatol Clin 1996; 14(3): 399-421. [http://dx.doi.org/10.1016/S0733-8635(05)70368-5] [PMID: 8818550]

[107] Gupta MA, Gupta AK. Psychodermatology: an update. J Am Acad Dermatol 1996; 34(6): 1030-46. [http://dx.doi.org/10.1016/S0190-9622(96)90284-4] [PMID: 8647969]

[108] Koblenzer CS. Psychosomatic concepts in dermatology. A dermatologist-psychoanalyst's viewpoint. Arch Dermatol 1983; 119(6): 501-12. [http://dx.doi.org/10.1001/archderm.1983.01650300055017] [PMID: 6859891]

[109] Anzieu D. Le moi-peau. Paris: Dunod 1985.

[110] Sifneos PE. The prevalence of 'alexithymic' characteristics in psychosomatic patients. Psychother Psychosom 1973; 22(2): 255-62. [http://dx.doi.org/10.1159/000286529] [PMID: 4770536]

[111] Marty P, De M'Uzan M. La pensée opératoire. Rev Fr Psychanal 1963; 17: 345-55.

[112] Slominski A, Mihm MC. Potential mechanism of skin response to stress. Int J Dermatol 1996; 35(12): 849-51. [http://dx.doi.org/10.1111/j.1365-4362.1996.tb05049.x] [PMID: 8970839]

[113] Walker CD, Bodnar M, Forget MA, Toufexis DJ, Trottier G. Stress et plasticité neuroendocrinienne. Med Sci (Paris) 1997; 13: 509-18. [http://dx.doi.org/10.4267/10608/406]

[114] Dhabhar FS. Stress-induced enhancement of cell-mediated immunity. Ann N Y Acad Sci 1998; 840: 359-72. [http://dx.doi.org/10.1111/j.1749-6632.1998.tb09575.x] [PMID: 9629263]

[115] Dhabhar FS, McEwen BS. Enhancing *versus* suppressive effects of stress hormones on skin immune function. Proc Natl Acad Sci USA 1999; 96(3): 1059-64. [http://dx.doi.org/10.1073/pnas.96.3.1059] [PMID: 9927693]

[116] Harbuz MS, Conde GL, Marti O, Lightman SL, Jessop DS. The hypothalamic-pituitary-adrenal axis in autoimmunity. Ann N Y Acad Sci 1997; 823: 214-24. [http://dx.doi.org/10.1111/j.1749-6632.1997.tb48393.x] [PMID: 9292047]

[117] Misery L, Rousset H. La pelade est-elle une maladie psychosomatique? Rev Med Interne 2001; 22(3): 274-9. [http://dx.doi.org/10.1016/S0248-8663(00)00328-3] [PMID: 11270270]

[118] Pavlovic S, Daniltchenko M, Tobin DJ, *et al.* Further exploring the brain-skin connection: stress

worsens dermatitis *via* substance P-dependent neurogenic inflammation in mice. J Invest Dermatol 2008; 128(2): 434-46.
[http://dx.doi.org/10.1038/sj.jid.5701079] [PMID: 17914449]

[119] Singh LK, Pang X, Alexacos N, Letourneau R, Theoharides TC. Acute immobilization stress triggers skin mast cell degranulation *via* corticotropin releasing hormone, neurotensin, and substance P: A link to neurogenic skin disorders. Brain Behav Immun 1999; 13(3): 225-39.
[http://dx.doi.org/10.1006/brbi.1998.0541] [PMID: 10469524]

[120] Saint-Mezard P, Chavagnac C, Bosset S, *et al.* Psychological stress exerts an adjuvant effect on skin dendritic cell functions *in vivo.* J Immunol 2003; 171(8): 4073-80.
[http://dx.doi.org/10.4049/jimmunol.171.8.4073] [PMID: 14530328]

[121] Nordlind K, Azmitia EC, Slominski A. The skin as a mirror of the soul: exploring the possible roles of serotonin. Exp Dermatol 2008; 17(4): 301-11.
[http://dx.doi.org/10.1111/j.1600-0625.2007.00670.x] [PMID: 18177349]

[122] Tausk FA, Nousari H. Stress and the skin. Arch Dermatol 2001; 137(1): 78-82.
[http://dx.doi.org/10.1001/archderm.137.1.78] [PMID: 11176665]

[123] Buske-Kirschbaum A, Hellhammer DH. Endocrine and immune responses to stress in chronic inflammatory skin disorders. Ann N Y Acad Sci 2003; 992: 231-40.
[http://dx.doi.org/10.1111/j.1749-6632.2003.tb03153.x] [PMID: 12794062]

[124] Slominski A, Wortsman J, Tuckey RC, Paus R. Differential expression of HPA axis homolog in the skin. Mol Cell Endocrinol 2007; 265-266: 143-9.
[http://dx.doi.org/10.1016/j.mce.2006.12.012] [PMID: 17197073]

[125] Misery L, Ständer S. Pruritus. London: Springer 2010.
[http://dx.doi.org/10.1007/978-1-84882-322-8]

[126] Misery L, Brenaut E, Le Garrec R, *et al.* Neuropathic pruritus. Nat Rev Neurol 2014; 10(7): 408-16.
[http://dx.doi.org/10.1038/nrneurol.2014.99] [PMID: 24912513]

[127] Yosipovitch G. The pruritus receptor unit: a target for novel therapies. J Invest Dermatol 2007; 127(8): 1857-9.
[http://dx.doi.org/10.1038/sj.jid.5700818] [PMID: 17632568]

[128] Schmelz M, Schmidt R, Bickel A, Handwerker HO, Torebjörk HE. Specific C-receptors for itch in human skin. J Neurosci 1997; 17(20): 8003-8.
[PMID: 9315918]

[129] Schmelz M, Schmidt R, Weidner C, Hilliges M, Torebjörk HE, Handwerker HO. Chemical response pattern of different classes of C-nociceptors to pruritogens and algogens. J Neurophysiol 2003; 89(5): 2441-8.
[http://dx.doi.org/10.1152/jn.01139.2002] [PMID: 12611975]

[130] Ikoma A, Steinhoff M, Ständer S, Yosipovitch G, Schmelz M. The neurobiology of itch. Nat Rev Neurosci 2006; 7(7): 535-47.
[http://dx.doi.org/10.1038/nrn1950] [PMID: 16791143]

[131] Johanek LM, Meyer RA, Friedman RM, *et al.* A role for polymodal C-fiber afferents in nonhistaminergic itch. J Neurosci 2008; 28(30): 7659-69.

[http://dx.doi.org/10.1523/JNEUROSCI.1760-08.2008] [PMID: 18650342]

[132] Steinhoff M, Neisius U, Ikoma A, *et al.* Proteinase-activated receptor-2 mediates itch: a novel pathway for pruritus in human skin. J Neurosci 2003; 23(15): 6176-80.
[PMID: 12867500]

[133] Sikand P, Shimada SG, Green BG, LaMotte RH. Sensory responses to injection and punctate application of capsaicin and histamine to the skin. Pain 2011; 152(11): 2485-94.
[http://dx.doi.org/10.1016/j.pain.2011.06.001] [PMID: 21802851]

[134] Akiyama T, Carstens E. Neural processing of itch. Neuroscience 2013; 250: 697-714.
[http://dx.doi.org/10.1016/j.neuroscience.2013.07.035] [PMID: 23891755]

[135] Andrew D, Craig AD. Spinothalamic lamina I neurons selectively sensitive to histamine: a central neural pathway for itch. Nat Neurosci 2001; 4(1): 72-7.
[http://dx.doi.org/10.1038/82924] [PMID: 11135647]

[136] Davidson S, Zhang X, Khasabov SG, *et al.* Pruriceptive spinothalamic tract neurons: physiological properties and projection targets in the primate. J Neurophysiol 2012; 108(6): 1711-23.
[http://dx.doi.org/10.1152/jn.00206.2012] [PMID: 22723676]

[137] Hsieh JC, Hägermark O, Ståhle-Bäckdahl M, *et al.* Urge to scratch represented in the human cerebral cortex during itch. J Neurophysiol 1994; 72(6): 3004-8.
[PMID: 7897505]

[138] Dhand A, Aminoff MJ. The neurology of itch. Brain 2014; 137(Pt 2): 313-22.
[http://dx.doi.org/10.1093/brain/awt158] [PMID: 23794605]

[139] Papoiu AD, Coghill RC, Kraft RA, Wang H, Yosipovitch G. A tale of two itches. Common features and notable differences in brain activation evoked by cowhage and histamine induced itch. Neuroimage 2012; 59(4): 3611-23.
[http://dx.doi.org/10.1016/j.neuroimage.2011.10.099] [PMID: 22100770]

[140] Suárez AL, Feramisco JD, Koo J, Steinhoff M. Psychoneuroimmunology of psychological stress and atopic dermatitis: pathophysiologic and therapeutic updates. Acta Derm Venereol 2012; 92(1): 7-15.
[http://dx.doi.org/10.2340/00015555-1188] [PMID: 22101513]

[141] Chrostowska-Plak D, Reich A, Szepietowski JC. Relationship between itch and psychological status of patients with atopic dermatitis. J Eur Acad Dermatol Venereol 2013; 27(2): e239-42.
[http://dx.doi.org/10.1111/j.1468-3083.2012.04578.x] [PMID: 22621673]

[142] Misery L, Chastaing M. Joint consultation by a psychiatrist and a dermatologist. Dermatol Psychosom 2003; 4: 160-4.
[http://dx.doi.org/10.1159/000073994]

CHAPTER 2

Psoriasis and Stress: A Review

Vera Leibovici[1,*] and **Alan Menter**[2]

[1] *Department of Dermatology Hadassah-Hebrew University Medical Center, Jerusalem, Israel*

[2] *Department of Dermatology, Baylor University Medical Center Dallas, TX, USA*

Abstract: Psoriasis is a chronic immune-mediated genetic disease affecting approximately 120 million patients worldwide. Over 40 genes are associated with psoriasis. Common trigger factors include infections, trauma, medications and stress. There is substantial literature describing the link between psychosocial stress and the exacerbation of psoriasis.

We conducted a comprehensive review of the literature regarding pathophysiology, personality traits, quality of life, anxiety, depression, sexual dysfunction, alcohol, smoking and the treatment of psoriasis with respect to stress.

Our understanding of the brain-skin axis may help alleviate the suffering of our psoriatic patient population and shed light on the pathophysiology of psoriasis.

Keywords: Anxiety, Depression, Pathophysiology, Personality trait psoriasis, Quality of life, Sexual dysfunction, Stress, Substance abuse, Treatment.

INTRODUCTION

Psoriasis is a chronic immune-mediated genetic disease affecting approximately 120 million patients worldwide. Over 40 genes are associated with psoriasis with common trigger factors including infections, trauma, medications and stress.

Stress has been described, as being an important exacerbating factor not only in psoriasis, but in many other dermatological diseases, such as atopic dermatitis,

* **Corresponding author Vera Leibovici:** Department of Dermatology Hadassah-Hebrew University Medical Center, Jerusalem 91120, Israel; Tel: 972-2-6776368; Fax: 972-2-6244801; E-mail: vleibovici@hadassah.org.il.

Klas Nordlind & Anna Zalewska-Janowska (Eds.)

acne vulgaris and chronic urticaria. Not all psoriatic patients believe that their disease is affected by stress: those who do are called "stress responders", as opposed to "non-stress responders" [1].

The literature depicts a range of 37%-78% of stress responders in psoriasis [2].

Living with psoriasis, a chronic, disfiguring disease, associated with social stigmata, poor self-esteem, anxiety and depression results in stress [3]. The stress in psoriasis can be generated by the disease itself or be caused by external psychosocial causes, such as bereavement, stress at work, family problems, financial matters, *etc.*

Kimball *et al.* [4] consider that the stress caused by living with psoriasis and psychosocial stress, that exacerbates psoriasis, is a bidirectional interaction that can even become a vicious cycle.

Psychosocial stress plays an important role in the exacerbation of psoriasis [5 - 8]. Gupta *et al.* [5] describe that the stress-responders have more severe psoriasis in the "emotionally charged" body areas, such as scalp, face, neck, forearms, hands and genital areas, while the total percentage of affected body surface does not vary. This is in line with the findings of Zachariae *et al.* [9], who also found that stress responders had more psoriatic lesions on the visible areas of the body rather than non-visible ones, while the total severity score (PASI) was not affected. However, Verhoeven *et al.* [10] endorsed a significant association between stress and severity of psoriasis. Fortune *et al.* [13] described that stress, apart from being a significant exacerbating factor for psoriasis can also affect the duration of treatment in psoriasis, (*e.g.,* stress-responders need more sustained therapies).

PATHOPHYSIOLOGY OF THE PSORIASIS- STRESS RELATIONSHIP

The underlying pathophysiological mechanisms by which psychosocial stress exacerbates psoriasis have been reviewed recently by Hunter *et al.* [14].

It can be explained by the link between the hypothalamo-pituitary adrenal (HPA) axis and the sympathetic nervous system (SNS), as well as by the release of nerve-related factors from peripheral sensory nerves. A peripheral HPA axis, which may "calibrate" the stress response of the central system has been found in the skin by several authors [15 - 18].

The nervous system pathway of the stress-psoriasis association has been suggested by Farber *et al.* and is supported by the fact that psoriasis has a symmetrical distribution and psoriatic lesions have been shown to sometimes resolve in areas of denervation [19, 20].

The nervous and immune systems are closely related and neuropeptides and neurotransmitters serve as a link between the systems. As discussed above, neuropeptides and neurotransmitters are released by nerves innervating the skin and influence mast cells and Langerhans cells located in close anatomical vicinity [21].

Psoriatic plaques in high stress group have increased nerve fiber density, altered content of neuropeptides, including calcitonin gene-related peptide (CGRP), substance P and nerve growth factor [22].

The role of mast cells in psoriasis has been reviewed by Harvima *et al.* [23]. Ark *et al.* [24] described that stress-related neuropeptides and neurotrophins, such as corticotropin-releasing hormone (CRH), substance P, CGRP, and nerve growth factor act also as mast cell secretagogues. The role of mast cells in stress-induced exacerbation of psoriasis has however, yet to be fully elucidated.

The stress-induced exacerbation of psoriasis through the HPA axis and the sympathetic adrenal–medullary system pathways (SAM) results in a defective adrenergic response.

Increased urinary epinephrine and decreased serum cortisol were found in psoriatic patients during stressor exposure, with lower baseline salivary and serum cortisol also found in stress-response psoriatic patients [25].

These results disagree with the findings of Buske-Kirschbaum *et al.* [26] using the dexamethasone suppression test, and Karanikas *et al.* [27] using the corticotropin releasing hormone (CRH) in order to stimulate the HPA axis, found little or no difference in the cortisol response between psoriatic patients and normal controls.

Under conditions of stress, the activation of the sympathetic nervous system may lead to an increase of the sympathetic neurotransmitter, norepinephrine and of the co-transmitter, adenosine-5-triphosphate with induction of IL-6 by endothelial cells, which might generate TH-17 cells [28].

The expression of CRH and CRH receptors (CRH-Rs) in the psoriatic involved skin is of high importance, due to their pro- and anti-inflammatory effects [29 - 31] with the literature showing conflicting results. Tagen *et al.* [32] and Zhou *et al.* [33] found reduced expression of CRH and CRH-Rs in the psoriatic involved skin, while O'Kane *et al.* [34] and Kono *et al.* [35] found their increased expression in the psoriatic skin.

The activation of sympathetic pathway, during stress, apart from a defective adrenergic response, may also cause an altered redistribution of leucocytes in the psoriatic skin.

Schmidt–Ott *et al.* [36] revealed that patients with psoriasis have increased circulating cutaneous lymphocyte-associated antigen (CLA) T cells and natural killer cells (NK). Since T cell activation precedes epidermal changes [37], this finding is likely of importance.

Buske-Kirschenbaum *et al.* [38] found raised circulating CD4+cells in psoriatic patients in response to stress. This finding is also of great relevance, since the infiltration of the skin with monocytes and CD4+ is an important part of the immunopathogenesis of psoriatic lesions [39].

PERSONALITY TRAITS IN PSORIASIS

Psoriasis being a chronic lifelong, relapsing disease with social stigmatization, can affect the personality of the patients.

Type D of personality encompasses a tendency for feeling negative emotions (anger, anxiety, or hostility) and a tendency for withdrawal from society. Basinka *et al.* [40] compared 90 psoriasis patients with 86 healthy controls, using DS-14 scale and found a more frequent occurrence of type D personality among psoriasis patients, especially increased negative affectivity. Zelyko-Penavic *et al.* [41] using Eysenk's Personal Questionnaire in 130 psoriatic patients found higher results on the psychoticism scale and lower results on the extroversion scale. Conversely,

Litaiem *et al.* [42] could not find any significant difference between temperament scores in 65 psoriasis patients and normal controls. Remrod *et al.* [43] demonstrated higher scores of SSP- embitterment, trait irritability, mistrust, and verbal trait aggression in early-onset psoriasis as compared to late-onset disease. These traits were seen by the authors as a consequence of long standing psoriasis and efforts to cope with it.

People with avoidant personality trait experience long-standing feelings of inadequacy and are extremely sensitive to what others think about them, leading them to be socially inhibited and feel socially inept. Magin *et al.* [44] studied 29 Australian patients psoriatic and found that they had avoidant personality traits.

According to Remrod *et al.* [45] psoriatic patients with severe pruritus differ psychologically from those with mild pruritus by presenting higher scores of personality traits, such as somatic trait anxiety, embitterment, mistrust, and physical trait aggression. Contrarily, Janowki *et al.* [46] could not reveal any significant association between pruritus and basic personality traits.

QUALITY OF LIFE IN PSORIASIS

Quality of life (QOL) in medicine reflects patients' subjective evaluation on the impact of disease on their physical, psychological and social functioning and well-being.

Quality of life instruments for psoriasis were reviewed in 2012 by Heller *et al.* [47]. According to the authors the useful QOL instruments are: Generic QoL instruments: Short Form 36, Sickness Impact Profile, General Health Questionnaire, Psychological General Well-Being Index.

Dermatology-specific QoL instruments are: Dermatology Life Quality Index, Dermatology Quality of Life Scales, Dermatology Specific Quality of Life, Skindex (Skindex-61, Skindex-29). Psoriasis-specific QoL instruments are: Psoriasis Disability Index, Psoriasis Life Stress Inventory, Psoriasis Index of Quality of Life, Salford Psoriasis Index, Psoriasis Quality of Life 12 items (a part of the Koo-Menter Psoriasis Instrument).

In Koo's population-based study of quality of life, the participants disclosed that

that they were concerned with two major issues: itching (pruritus) and appearance (body-image) [48].

Pruritus in psoriasis is more frequent than previously believed [49 - 53].The intensity of pruritus in psoriasis depends on the severity of depression and stigmatization [54]. Depression was found to modulate pruritus perception [54]. Psoriatic patients with severe pruritus differ psychologically from those with mild pruritus presenting higher scores of depression [45]. Pruritus can cause concentration difficulties, change in eating habits and sexual dysfunction [49] and can interfere with the ability to work [55].

Vulvar psoriasis causes itching that substantially affects patients' psychosocial well-being [56].

Psoriatic patients feel disfigured, and have a low self-esteem and self-confidence [48, 57]. The altered body image may result in further extension of body coverage, sexual inhibition, and reduced exercise activity [58].

The localization of the psoriatic lesions has an important impact on psoriasis patients' physical and mental health. This can be even more important than the clinical severity of the disease, which was found to affect minimally the quality of life of psoriatic patients [59].

Localization on visible areas the face, scalp, and hands are unattractive to the patients [60] and patients perceive the diseases more disabling [61, 62]. Localization on the palms and soles results in pain and discomfort and physical disability [63]. Nail involvement, that affects up to 60% of the psoriatic patients, can limit daily activities and cause psychological stress as well [64]. Palmoplantar psoriasis, pustular psoriasis or psoriatic arthritis are forms of psoriasis that have the most significant impairment of quality of life [65]. Psoriatic arthritis, frequently painful, confers the patients a significantly worse quality of life than of psoriasis without joint involvement [66, 67]. Contrarily, Fortune *et al.* believe that anatomical localization has only a modest association with patients' mental health [68].

Psychological functioning in psoriasis comprises impaired general mental health (anxiety, depression, loss of behavioral or emotional control and psychological well-being) and emotional reactions such as shame, embarrassment, self-consciousness, anger, helplessness [69].

Anxiety and depression in psoriasis are described in paragraphs 5 and 6.

Sleep might be adversely affected in psoriasis [49].This is most likely secondary to depression rather than related to a direct effect of psoriasis [70]. Conversely, other authors could not find sleep disturbances in a group of Italian psoriatic patients [71].

Psoriasis patients experience reduced well- being [72]. Psoriatic patients have a more passive attitude towards life and have lesser personal involvement with people and in addition they experience a higher feel loss of meaning in life compared with both atopic dermatitis and normal controls [72].

People with psoriasis feel embarrassed, helpless and self-conscious, due to the visibility of their disfiguring disease and their altered body image.

Psoriasis patients experience higher levels of stigmatization than do other dermatological patients [73]. Stigmatization strongly affects the physical and especially the mental health in psoriatic patients [74]. The level of stigmatization correlates with the level of pruritus, prior stress and depression [75].

Patient's illness perceptions are predictors of functional status in psoriasis [76].

Psoriatic patients anticipate other people negative reactions to their psoriasis, which contributes highly to their disability in everyday life [68].

Coping efforts in psoriasis are low. Mechanisms such as public avoidance, over-eating, alcohol abuse and smoking have a direct negative effect by exacerbating obesity and cardiac diseases [77]. Hence the adverse mental health aspects of psoriasis can have a direct effect or potentially worsen the diseases process [78]. Better coping mechanisms produce higher levels of mental health [79]. Higher levels of optimism were correlated with higher acceptance of disease in psoriatic patients [80].

Social functioning encompasses social activities, sexual behavior, personal relationships, work and career.

The visibility of the psoriatic lesions leads to overt public rejection experiences, such as being asked to leave a swimming pool, gym or hairdressers [81].

As a result of stigmatization patients avoid interpersonal relationships, which interferes with the sexual relations as well. Sexual dysfunction in psoriasis is described in paragraph 7.

Regarding family relationships psoriatic patients with lower levels of quality of life had partners with higher levels of depressive and anxious symptoms [82]. Family members of psoriatic patients also complain that their close relationship has been deteriorated [83].

Psoriatic patients have reduced occupational opportunities and earn less money and suffer from financial distress [61].

A small percentage (6%) of patients with severe psoriasis complain of work-place discrimination [63] and others recognize that psoriasis affected their choice of career [84].

The time and money spent on the treatment of severe psoriasis, becomes a financial burden and can affect the work status of psoriatic patients [83, 85], causing a higher rate of unemployment in the psoriasis population [68].

The social stigma of psoriasis decreases after mid-life when people are more established financially and socially [86, 87].

Psoriatic patients are frequently dissatisfied with the doctor–patient relationship. More than half of the patients emphasized their need to be listened to by the treating physician, and their wish that the physician should use simple language and improve their psychological skills and interpersonal communication techniques [88].

PSORIASIS AND ANXIETY

Anxiety is defined by the fifth edition of the diagnostic and statistical manual of mental disorders (DSM-5) as an excessive fear (emotional response to real or perceived imminent threat) and anxiety (anticipation of future threat). The fear or anxiety must last at least 6 months, cause significant distress or impairment in social life and may not be better explained by other mental disorders [89].

Psoriatic patients have been shown to have higher rates of anxiety than patients with cancer [90]. Social anxiety/avoidance is higher in psoriatic patients as compared to atopic dermatitis, contact dermatitis, acne and vitiligo [91].

Anxiety in psoriasis encompasses pathological worrying and social anxiety, such as avoidance, fears of negative evaluation and stigmatization [44, 92, 93]. Being unemployed was associated with a high likelihood of anxiety [94, 95]. Completion of graduate studies was considered to also be another factor related to anxiety [96].

There is a contradictory data in the literature on the relationship between psoriasis and anxiety. Rieder *et al.* [97] in a large review substantiated that these conflicting results are due to the lack of distinction made by the authors between the actual DSM diagnosis of generalized anxiety and subjective stress.

Richards *et al.* [98] found out an anxiety of 43% in psoriatic outpatients at a tertiary hospital. Similar results were found by Consoli *et al.* [99], Karanikas *et al.* [27], Zelyko *et al.* [41], Taner *et al.* [100] found only "mild anxiety" in psoriatic patients. However, Devrimci-Ozguven *et al.* [101] and Kilic *et al.* [102], in their studies were unable to find a link between psoriasis and anxiety.

Kurd *et al.* [103] in a large population-based study from the United Kingdom hypothesized that psoriasis confers 7100 diagnoses of anxiety each year (*e.g.* incidence of 0.011%).

The extent of skin involvement in many studies did not appear to relate to the degree of anxiety in psoriasis patients [95, 97, 103]. Contrarily, Pujol *et al.* [96] found in a multicenter study of 1164 Spanish psoriatic patients that reduction in disease severity improved anxiety. Schneider *et al.* [93] also found a correlation between social fear/avoidance and disease severity.

Anxiety has been shown to be higher in psoriatic arthritis than in psoriasis without arthritis [94, 95, 104 - 106].

Regarding the gender, female psoriatic patients were found to be more anxious [94, 95].

According to Remrod *et al.* [43] early-onset psoriatic patients were more anxious than late onset psoriasis. Conversely, Kotruya *et al.* [107] could not detect any differences relating to anxiety between early and late onset of psoriasis as well as the control group.

According to Remrod *et al.* [45] psoriatic patients with severe pruritus differ psychologically from those with mild pruritus by presenting higher scores of anxiety.

Fortune *et al.* described that anxiety negatively affects response to treatment, such as photochemotherapy [13]

Therapeutic modalities may also play a role in anxiety in psoriasis patients. Saraceno *et al.* [108], for instance found, that 4% of 141 psoriatic patients experienced panic attacks during treatment with infliximab an intravenous therapy given over a 1-2 hour time period.

Treatment with biological agents have given controversial effects on the anxiety of psoriatic arthritis patients. While Freire *et al.* [94] found that biological agents as monotherapy, or in combination with anti-rheumatic drugs improved anxiety in psoriatic arthritis patients, McDonought *et al.* [95] was unable to recognize such an improvement.

Dauden *et al.* [109] reported improved quality of life and anxiety in moderate –to-severe psoriasis receiving continuous etanacerpt, an anti-TNF biological treatment, for 52 weeks, as did Menter.

Menter *et al.* [110] reported improvement in quality of life and anxiety in psoriatic patients receiving adalimumab.

In addition, Ustekinumab, a human anti-interleukin-12/23 monoclonal antibody was also shown to improve also anxiety in psoriasis patients [111].

It is thus highly important that dermatologists and other physicians make the correct diagnosis and treat anxiety appropriately in psoriasis in order to improve the quality of life of each and every patient.

PSORIASIS AND DEPRESSION

Depression is described in the fifth edition of the diagnostic and statistical manual of mental disorders (DSM-5) as the presence of sad, empty or irritable mood, accompanied by somatic and cognitive changes that significantly affect the individual's capacity to function. DSM-5 classifies depression into disruptive mood dysregulation disorder, major depressive disorder, persistent depressive disorder (dysthymia), premenstrual dysphoric disorder, substance/medication-induced depressive disorder and depressive disorder due to another medical condition [112].

Gupta *et al.* [117] found a greater percentage of psoriatic patients suffering from depression than in patients with acne, alopecia areata, atopic dermatitis, while Akay *et al.* [114] demonstrated a higher depression rate in patients with psoriasis as compared to lichen planus.

In a critical review of 98 studies of psoriasis and depression, published up to 2014, Dowlatshahi *et al.* [115] concluded that population-based studies showed an incidence of at least one and a half times more depression in psoriasis than in the normal population. They also stated that 2-10% of psoriasis patients from the general population suffer from clinical depression and 20-25% have depressive symptoms [115]. Suicidal ideation in psoriasis ranges between 1.44-8.6% and is seen more commonly in younger patients [103, 113, 116].

Depression in psoriasis is likely caused by the impaired quality of life, in addition to the common inflammatory mediators implicated in both diseases.

The detrimental body image of psoriatic patients, leading to stigmatization, their difficulties in establishing social and interpersonal relationships, such as inter-personal anxiety, along with shame, embarrassment and isolation leads to depression, anxiety and even suicidal ideation [103, 104, 117, 118]. Several authors reported that that the perception of stigmatization was the most significant factor in predicting depression on psoriasis [98, 104, 117]. Regarding external stress factors that precipitated depression and anxiety in psoriasis, unemployment was found to be the strongest factor [95].

Psoriasis and depression have common inflammatory mediators, including tumor necrosing factor (TNF alpha) and interferon-gamma, both important cytokines in the pathogenesis of both diseases [119, 120]. This might be a plausible, but still unproven, explanation of the high association of psoriasis and depression. Whether either or both of these mediators play a significant role in depression in the psoriasis population still remains to be fully determined as to date the vast majority of the studies have found no relationship between depression in psoriasis and disease severity [49, 98, 104, 121].

Likewise, there does not appear to be a correlation between mean-age, gender of psoriatic patients and depression [97]. Kurd *et al.*, however did reveal a higher risk of depression in men and younger psoriasis patients [103].

A higher rate of depression in psoriatic arthritis, as compared to psoriasis alone has been reported by several authors [94, 95, 105, 106]. The severity of depression in psoriatic arthritis was dependent on the higher number of actively inflamed joints [121]. Other authors [114, 122 - 124] however, have not found this relationship between depression and psoriatic arthritis.

According to Kotruya *et al.* [107], patients with late-onset psoriasis had more prominent symptoms of depression compared with the group of early-onset psoriasis. Conversely, Remrod *et al.* [43] found that early onset psoriasis was associated with significantly more depressed patients than late-onset psoriasis.

Pruritus intensity in psoriasis is associated with psychological factors, such as depression. According to Remrod *et al.* [45] psoriatic patients with severe pruritus differ psychologically from those with mild pruritus by presenting higher scores of depression.

Several studies have revealed a relationship between depression and sexual dysfunction [125 - 127]. Emerctan [128] on the contrary did not find such a relationship. Mercan *et al.* [125] noted that patients with psoriasis had problems specifically relating to orgasm and not to sexual drive. The authors concluded that the sexual dysfunction found in their patients might be due to other factors rather than depression.

Multiple medications used for the treatment of psoriasis have been implicated in causing depression. Depression was induced by etretinate in 3 cases [129].

In addition, two patients committed suicide while receiving adalimumab. One of the patients had a psychiatric background [130]. This is a rare occurrence as the vast majority of patients with moderate to severe psoriasis, have shown significant benefit from adalimumab in improving their depression [110]. Etanercept and infliximab, two other biological treatments that affect tumor necrosis factor, have also been reported to improve depression in psoriatic patients [131, 132] as Ustekinumab, a human anti-interleukin-12/23 monoclonal antibody [111]. These findings substantiate the hypothesis that psoriasis and depression are likely bound by common inflammatory mediators.

PSORIASIS AND SEXUAL DYSFUNCTION

Sexual dysfunction has been described in many chronic skin conditions associated with psychological impairment such as vitiligo [133, 134] chronic urticaria [134] and atopic dermatitis [125, 128].

The first to describe sexual dysfunction in psoriatic patients were Gupta *et al.* [127], who reported no significant relationship between marital status, age, gender and duration of psoriasis and sexual problems encountered by the patients

The disruptive impact of psoriasis on patients' sexual functioning has been reported by many others [125, 126, 128, 135 - 137]. Sexual dysfunction is caused by two factors: psychological and organic. Psychological factors in psoriasis include anxiety, depression, detrimental body image, difficulties in establishing social and interpersonal relationships, such as interpersonal anxiety, along with shame and embarrassment [138].

Organic factors include erectile dysfunction in men and female sexual functions. Psoriatic male patients have a higher prevalence of erectile dysfunction [128, 139, 140]. Conversely, Goulding [141] believes that psoriasis is not a risk factor for erectile dysfunction in men. Impaired female sexual functions were also found in psoriatic women [121, 140].

Erectile dysfunction in men may be caused by pelvic arterial atherosclerosis, which is considered a predictor of future cardiovascular disease, seen in higher frequency in the psoriasis population.

In 2012, Kurizky *et al.* [142] published a systematic review of sexual dysfunction in patients with psoriasis and psoriatic arthritis, revealing that the literature on this subject is scarce, and emphasize the need for further investigations.

Sampogna *et al.* [126] and Guenther *et al.* [137] found that severe and moderate psoriasis were more associated with sexual dysfunction. Contrarily, Emerctan *et al.* [128] and Al-Mazeedi *et al.* [135] could not find any relationship between the severity of psoriasis and sexual dysfunction.

Regarding the localization of psoriasis, the presence of genital psoriasis was found to have an impact on sexual dysfunction, only in women [136]. This is of importance, since 48.8% of male psoriatic patients and 32.7% of female psoriatic patients suffer from genital involvement [143]. Molina-Leyva *et al.* [144] revealed that psoriasis lesions on abdomen, genitals, lumbar region and buttocks in women and chest, genitals and buttocks in men were associated with increased sexual dysfunction. No relationship between genital psoriasis and sexual dysfunction could be found by others [126, 128].

Patients with psoriatic arthritis have reduced physical activity, more fatigue and present with higher rates of anxiety and depression than patients with psoriasis without joint involvement [95]. The impaired quality of life in psoriatic arthritis can aggravate sexual dysfunction as well [126, 127].

While several studies revealed a positive relationship between depression and sexual dysfunction [126, 127], Emerctan found no such relationship [128]. Mercan *et al.* [125] have noticed that patients with psoriasis had problems with orgasm and not sexual drive. Since depression is related especially to sexual drive, the authors conclude that the sexual dysfunction found in their patients might be due to other factors rather than depression.

Psoriasis therapeutic agents may also play a role in altering sexual function. Methotrexate can, on occasion, cause reduced libido and erectile dysfunction [145] or sexual impotence [146]. Etretinate was also described to produce erectile dysfunction [147].

Two anti-TNF biological treatments, etanacerpt and adalimumab have been shown to improve sexual dysfunction in psoriasis, *i.e.* the index of erectile functions in men and sexual index function in females [140]. Ustekinumab, a human anti-interleukin-12/23 monoclonal antibody also improved sexual dysfunction in a large clinical trial [137]. Further studies are needed in order to elucidate the organic etiology of sexual dysfunction in psoriasis.

A study of 400 patients in press (JAAD) from Dublin, Ireland (Brian Kirby) and Dallas, USA, (Caitriona Ryan and Alan Menter) has also shown significant clinical evidence of genital psoriasis involvement (up to 60%) with associated sexual activity quality of life improvements.

PSORIASIS AND SMOKING

In a systemic review and meta-analysis, Amstrong *et al.* [148] concluded that smoking is an independent risk factor for the development of psoriasis and that patients with established psoriasis continue to smoke more than patients without psoriasis.

Setty *et al.* [149] revealed in a prospective study that the risk of developing psoriasis in women was higher not only for current smokers, but also for past smokers, the risk decreasing with each year of cessation. Passive smoking was found out to be also a risk factor for psoriasis [12]. Smoking was encountered more commonly in patients with pustular psoriasis [11].

The pathways whereby smoking exacerbates psoriasis are driven either through a nicotinic receptor mediated pathway [150], or through T-cell activation and inflammatory cytokines, such as TNF-alpha [149, 150]. It is well known that smoking is a risk factor for myocardial infarction in the non-psoriasis population. In addition, there is also a definite cardiovascular risk in patients with moderate to severe as well as early-onset psoriasis [151, 152] thus, making smoking an additional problem in the psoriasis population.

Patients with psoriasis also have a higher risk of metabolic syndrome (obesity, hypertension, diabetes mellitus and dyslipidemia), thus further exacerbating the coronary artery risk issue in these patients [152].

Smoking in psoriasis was found to cause only a small increased risk for cancer of lung and urinary bladder [153].

Psoriasis is a significant emotional burden for patients from an early age and smoking, as well as alcoholism is considered to be a coping mechanism in this stigmatizing disease [154, 155].

People smoke in order to relieve anxious and psychotic disorders, so smoking is a potential confounder not only in psoriasis, but in other psycho-cutaneous diseases.

Menter *et al.* [156], on behalf of the International Psoriasis Foundation, recommend lifestyle modification plans in psoriatic patients, including the limitation of alcohol and tobacco intake, which has the potential to not only benefit their general medical health but also their psoriasis.

PSORIASIS AND ALCOHOL INTAKE

The relationship between psoriasis and alcohol intake is complex and controversial. It is still unclear whether alcohol intake is a true risk factor of psoriasis or an epiphenomenon of coping with the distress caused by the disease. Most authors depicted an association between alcohol intake and psoriasis [12, 154, 155, 157 - 159] while others did not [160, 161], due possibly to the different ways of reporting alcohol consumption [97].

Alcohol is secreted in skin, has a negative impact on the immune system and stimulates keratinocyte proliferation *in vitro* [10]. Skin alcohol can enhance cytokine production, and enhance lymphocyte proliferation, *in vitro* [162 - 164].

Alcohol consumption in psoriatic patients was associated with greater severity of the disease [165, 166].

Heavy drinkers present with a different clinical picture of psoriasis, which might be either very inflamed with mild scaling, or hyperkeratotic plaques [165, 167].

Excessive alcohol consumption may contribute to systemic inflammation, aggravating cardiovascular diseases and depression, which are comorbidities of psoriasis [168]. Kirby *et al.* [169] also consider that psoriatic patients who consume alcohol exhibit more psychiatric morbidity, such as anxiety and depression.

The risk of mortality in moderate to severe psoriasis patients is increased by alcohol consumption [170]. In alcoholic patients anti-psoriatic treatment are less effective, more toxic and the patients are less compliant [162]. Likewise, alcohol moderation is essential in patients on methotrexate therapy, to reduce liver toxicity.

The literature emphases the pharmacological interactions between psoriatic drugs and alcohol intake. Thus, red wine reduces the efficacy of cyclosporine [171], while heavy alcohol intake increases levels of cyclosporine in the blood [172]. Ethanol contributes to the conversion of acitretin to etretinate, thus precluding its use in females of child-bearing potential [173].

Alcohol intake in psoriasis may be also regarded as a self-relieving medication, in order to cope with the stress induced by the disease [97].

Risk factor, or epiphenomenon, the role of alcohol in psoriasis is detrimental and needs further elucidation.

TREATMENT OF STRESS IN PSORIASIS

Psoriasis is a 'brain-skin axis' disease [1]. In previous chapters, we have shown that many psoriatic patients are more susceptible to stress than others("stress-responders") and that psoriatic patients, are more prone to develop psychiatric diseases than patients with other dermatological diseases.

In one study, clearance of psoriasis after standard treatments, did not impact patients' psychological distress, and their beliefs about psoriasis or on coping with the disease [174]. This observation highlights the need for complementary specific treatment to improve stress reduction in these patients. On the contrary, psoriatic patients receiving anti-TNF-alpha biological treatment (etanercept, infliximab and adalimumab) showed improvement in well-being, anxiety and depression scores [109, 110, 132]. Similar effects have also been noted with ustekimumab, an anti-interleukin12/23 monoclonal antibody [111].

Treatment of stress in psoriatic patients can be divided into two main categories: Psychotherapy and Pharmacotherapy.

In a 2013 review of the literature, Fordham *et al.* [175] concluded that existing studies are insufficient to judge whether reduction interventions in psoriasis are effective.

Behavioral therapies used in psoriasis include relaxation therapy, hypnosis and biofeedback. Relaxation therapies affect the autonomic nervous system and the immune system, thus improving psoriasis [176]. Hypnosis and biofeedback have been used in psoriasis patients with beneficial results [177, 178]. Hypnosis may also enhance the effects obtained by biofeedback [179]. Thermal biofeedback was used in one patient with success [180].

Various forms of cognitive -behavior therapy (CBT) have been used in the treatment of psoriasis. A combination of relaxation and cognitive techniques has been shown to reduce anxiety and self-reported severity scale in a study of 11 patients [181]. Fortune *et al.* used a cognitive –behavioral symptom management programme (PSMP) as an adjuvant in psoriasis therapy and found a reduction in clinical severity of psoriasis, as well as in anxiety, depression and psoriasis-related stress [182]. PSMP was found to have no effect on self-reported coping strategies [183].

Mindfulness based cognitive therapy (MBCT) aims to reduce psychological distress by developing non-judgmental awareness of the present moment and of acceptance of the demands of daily life [184]. In a pilot study, psoriatic patients receiving MBCT as an adjuvant therapy reported lower psoriasis severity score and quality of life impairment, but no improvement in their perceived stress [185]. Mindfulness based stress reduction tapes during phototherapy received by psoriatic patients accelerated the time to clearance [186, 187]. Online CBT, a web-based psychological intervention, showed improvement in anxiety and quality of life, but not in depression in psoriatic patients [188].

Self-help psychological approaches have the potential to relieve the psychosocial burden and relieve distress associated with disfigurement in psoriasis [189 - 191].

Psychotherapy has been used by Ulnik in a number of psoriatic patients with promising results [192].

The first-line pharmacological therapy in stress reduction of psoriatic patients who are non-depressed stress-responders, are the agents such as fluoxetine, paroxetine, sertraline or escitalopram [3]. Paroxetine is preferential because of its anti-anxiety effect and its less anti-cholinergic activity than the other SSRI's, with no weight gain. They also recommend anti-anxiety medication, such as alprazolam for only short-term, due to their potential to be addictive and highly sedative when used for longer periods [3].

Regarding mild-moderate depression in psoriasis, SSRI's should also be the first line treatment, being less cardiotoxic than tricyclic antidepressants [193]. Escitalopram, an SSRI, improved perceived symptom severity, quality of life and adherence to the treatment in patients suffering from psoriasis and depression [194].

All three TNF-alpha inhibitory agents, Adalimumab, Etanercept, and Infliximab were found to improve depression in psoriasis [109, 110, 132]. Ustekinumab, a human anti-interleukin-12/23 monoclonal antibody also substantially improved depression and anxiety in psoriatic patients [111].

CONCLUSION

It is imperative that dermatologists and all allied health professionals involved in the care of patients with psoriasis play a significant role in deterring the degree of stress, anxiety, and depression in each and every patient. In this paper we have reviewed the pathophysiology of psoriasis-stress relationship, in addition to the literature on all aspects of quality of life and psychiatric comorbidities in this population group with appropriate therapeutic options to ensure that all psoriasis patients live as normal of life as possible, both physical and emotionally .

Advisory Board: AbbVie, Allergan, Amgen, Boehringer Ingelheim, Eli –Lilly, Genentech, Janssen, Leo Pharma, Pfizer

Consultant: Abbvie, Allergan, Amgen, Convoy Therapeutics, Eli-Lilly, Janssen, Leo Pharma, Novartis, Pfizer, Syntrix, Vitae, XenoPort

Investigator: AbbVie, Allergan, Amgen, Boehringer Ingelheim, Celgene, Eli-Lilly,Genentech,Janssen,LeoPharma, erck,Novartis,Pfizer, Symbio/Maruho, Syntrix, Wyeth

Compension:(grant or honoraria): Abbvie, Allergan, Amgen, Boehringer Ingelheim, Celgene, Convoy Therapeutics, Eli-Lilly, Genentech, Janssen, LeoPharma , Merk, Novartis, Pfizer, Symbio/Maruho, Syntrix, Vitae,Wyeth, XenoPort

CONFLICT OF INTEREST

The authors confirm that they have no conflict of interest to declare for this publication.

ACKNOWLEDGEMENTS

Declared none.

REFERENCES

[1] Koo JY. Psychodermatology: a practical manual for clinicians. Curr Probl Dermatol 1995; 6: 204-32. [http://dx.doi.org/10.1016/S1040-0486(09)80012-4]

[2] Picardi A, Abeni D. Stressful life events and skin diseases: disentangling evidence from myth. Psychother Psychosom 2001; 70(3): 118-36. [http://dx.doi.org/10.1159/000056237] [PMID: 11340413]

[3] Heller MM, Lee ES, Koo JY. Stress as an influencing factor in psoriasis. Skin Therapy Lett 2011; 16(5): 1-4. [PMID: 21611682]

[4] Kimball AB, Jacobson C, Weiss S, Vreeland MG, Wu Y. The psychosocial burden of psoriasis. Am J Clin Dermatol 2005; 6(6): 383-92. [http://dx.doi.org/10.2165/00128071-200506060-00005] [PMID: 16343026]

[5] Gupta MA, Gupta AK, Kirkby S, *et al.* A psychocutaneous profile of psoriasis patients who are stress reactors. A study of 127 patients. Gen Hosp Psychiatry 1989; 11(3): 166-73. [http://dx.doi.org/10.1016/0163-8343(89)90036-4] [PMID: 2721939]

[6] Rigopoulos D, Gregoriou S, Katrinaki A, *et al.* Characteristics of psoriasis in Greece: an epidemiological study of a population in a sunny Mediterranean climate. Eur J Dermatol 2010; 20(2):

189-95.
[PMID: 20123642]

[7] Seville RH. Psoriasis and stress. Br J Dermatol 1977; 97(3): 297-302.
[http://dx.doi.org/10.1111/j.1365-2133.1977.tb15186.x] [PMID: 921900]

[8] Al'Abadie MS, Kent GG, Gawkrodger DJ. The relationship between stress and the onset and exacerbation of psoriasis and other skin conditions. Br J Dermatol 1994; 130(2): 199-203.
[http://dx.doi.org/10.1111/j.1365-2133.1994.tb02900.x] [PMID: 8123572]

[9] Zachariae R, Zachariae H, Blomqvist K, *et al.* Self-reported stress reactivity and psoriasis-related stress of Nordic psoriasis sufferers. J Eur Acad Dermatol Venereol 2004; 18(1): 27-36.
[http://dx.doi.org/10.1111/j.1468-3083.2004.00721.x] [PMID: 14678528]

[10] Verhoeven EW, Kraaimaat FW, de Jong EM, Schalkwijk J, van de Kerkhof PC, Evers AW. Individual differences in the effect of daily stressors on psoriasis: a prospective study. Br J Dermatol 2009; 161(2): 295-9.
[http://dx.doi.org/10.1111/j.1365-2133.2009.09194.x] [PMID: 19438455]

[11] Naldi L, Chatenoud L, Linder D, *et al.* Cigarette smoking, body mass index, and stressful life events as risk factors for psoriasis: results from an Italian case-control study. J Invest Dermatol 2005; 125(1): 61-7.
[http://dx.doi.org/10.1111/j.0022-202X.2005.23681.x] [PMID: 15982303]

[12] Jankovic S, Raznatovic M, Marinkovic J, Jankovic J, Maksimovic N. Risk factors for psoriasis: A case-control study. J Dermatol 2009; 36(6): 328-34.
[http://dx.doi.org/10.1111/j.1346-8138.2009.00648.x] [PMID: 19500181]

[13] Fortune DG, Richards HL, Kirby B, *et al.* Psychological distress impairs clearance of psoriasis in patients treated with photochemotherapy. Arch Dermatol 2003; 139(6): 752-6.
[http://dx.doi.org/10.1001/archderm.139.6.752] [PMID: 12810506]

[14] Hunter HJ, Griffiths CE, Kleyn CE. Does psychosocial stress play a role in the exacerbation of psoriasis? Br J Dermatol 2013; 169(5): 965-74.
[http://dx.doi.org/10.1111/bjd.12478] [PMID: 23796214]

[15] Slominski A, Wortsman J, Luger T, Paus R, Solomon S. Corticotropin releasing hormone and proopiomelanocortin involvement in the cutaneous response to stress. Physiol Rev 2000; 80(3): 979-1020.
[PMID: 10893429]

[16] Zmijewski MA, Slominski AT. Neuroendocrinology of the skin: An overview and selective analysis. Dermatoendocrinol 2011; 3(1): 3-10.
[http://dx.doi.org/10.4161/derm.3.1.14617] [PMID: 21519402]

[17] Ito N, Ito T, Kromminga A, *et al.* Human hair follicles display a functional equivalent of the hypothalamic-pituitary-adrenal axis and synthesize cortisol. FASEB J 2005; 19(10): 1332-4.
[PMID: 15946990]

[18] Arnetz BB, Fjellner B, Eneroth P, Kallner A. Stress and psoriasis: psychoendocrine and metabolic reactions in psoriatic patients during standardized stressor exposure. Psychosom Med 1985; 47(6): 528-41.

[http://dx.doi.org/10.1097/00006842-198511000-00003] [PMID: 4070523]

[19] Farber EM, Lanigan SW, Boer J. The role of cutaneous sensory nerves in the maintenance of psoriasis. Int J Dermatol 1990; 29(6): 418-20.
[http://dx.doi.org/10.1111/j.1365-4362.1990.tb03825.x] [PMID: 2397964]

[20] Farber EM, Nickoloff BJ, Recht B, Fraki JE. Stress, symmetry, and psoriasis: possible role of neuropeptides. J Am Acad Dermatol 1986; 14(2 Pt 1): 305-11.
[http://dx.doi.org/10.1016/S0190-9622(86)70034-0] [PMID: 2419375]

[21] Madva EN, Granstein RD. Nerve-derived transmitters including peptides influence cutaneous immunology. Brain Behav Immun 2013; 34: 1-10.
[http://dx.doi.org/10.1016/j.bbi.2013.03.006] [PMID: 23517710]

[22] Reich A, Orda A, Wiśnicka B, Szepietowski JC. Plasma concentration of selected neuropeptides in patients suffering from psoriasis. Exp Dermatol 2007; 16(5): 421-8.
[http://dx.doi.org/10.1111/j.1600-0625.2007.00544.x] [PMID: 17437485]

[23] Harvima IT, Nilsson G, Suttle MM, Naukkarinen A. Is there a role for mast cells in psoriasis? Arch Dermatol Res 2008; 300(9): 461-78.
[http://dx.doi.org/10.1007/s00403-008-0874-x] [PMID: 18719932]

[24] Arck PC, Slominski A, Theoharides TC, Peters EM, Paus R. Neuroimmunology of stress: skin takes center stage. J Invest Dermatol 2006; 126(8): 1697-704.
[http://dx.doi.org/10.1038/sj.jid.5700104] [PMID: 16845409]

[25] Richards HL, Ray DW, Kirby B, *et al.* Response of the hypothalamic-pituitary-adrenal axis to psychological stress in patients with psoriasis. Br J Dermatol 2005; 153(6): 1114-20.
[http://dx.doi.org/10.1111/j.1365-2133.2005.06817.x] [PMID: 16307645]

[26] Buske-Kirschbaum A, Ebrecht M, Kern S, Hellhammer DH. Endocrine stress responses in TH1-mediated chronic inflammatory skin disease (psoriasis vulgaris)--do they parallel stress-induced endocrine changes in TH2-mediated inflammatory dermatoses (atopic dermatitis)? Psychoneuroendocrinology 2006; 31(4): 439-46.
[http://dx.doi.org/10.1016/j.psyneuen.2005.10.006] [PMID: 16359823]

[27] Karanikas E, Harsoulis F, Giouzepas I, Griveas I. Stimulation of the hypothalamic-pituitary-adrenal axis with corticotropin releasing hormone in patients with psoriasis. Hormones (Athens) 2007; 6(4): 314-20.
[http://dx.doi.org/10.14310/horm.2002.1111027] [PMID: 18055422]

[28] Stohl LL, Zang JB, Ding W, Manni M, Zhou XK, Granstein RD. Norepinephrine and adenosine-5--triphosphate synergize in inducing IL-6 production by human dermal microvascular endothelial cells. Cytokine 2013; 64(2): 605-12.
[http://dx.doi.org/10.1016/j.cyto.2013.08.005] [PMID: 24026137]

[29] Theoharides TC, Cochrane DE. Critical role of mast cells in inflammatory diseases and the effect of acute stress. J Neuroimmunol 2004; 146(1-2): 1-12.
[http://dx.doi.org/10.1016/j.jneuroim.2003.10.041] [PMID: 14698841]

[30] Correa SG, Riera CM, Spiess J, Bianco ID. Modulation of the inflammatory response by corticotropin-releasing factor. Eur J Pharmacol 1997; 319(1): 85-90.

[http://dx.doi.org/10.1016/S0014-2999(96)00824-2] [PMID: 9030902]

[31] Thomas HA, Ling N, Wei ET. CRF and related peptides as anti-inflammatory agonists. Ann N Y Acad Sci 1993; 697: 219-28.
[http://dx.doi.org/10.1111/j.1749-6632.1993.tb49934.x] [PMID: 8257011]

[32] Tagen M, Stiles L, Kalogeromitros D, *et al.* Skin corticotropin-releasing hormone receptor expression in psoriasis. J Invest Dermatol 2007; 127(7): 1789-91.
[http://dx.doi.org/10.1038/sj.jid.5700757] [PMID: 17330132]

[33] Zhou C, Yu X, Cai D, Liu C, Li C. Role of corticotropin-releasing hormone and receptor in the pathogenesis of psoriasis. Med Hypotheses 2009; 73(4): 513-5.
[http://dx.doi.org/10.1016/j.mehy.2009.02.051] [PMID: 19560286]

[34] O'Kane M, Murphy EP, Kirby B. The role of corticotropin-releasing hormone in immune-mediated cutaneous inflammatory disease. Exp Dermatol 2006; 15(3): 143-53.
[http://dx.doi.org/10.1111/j.1600-0625.2006.00382.x] [PMID: 16480421]

[35] Kono M, Nagata H, Umemura S, Kawana S, Osamura RY. In situ expression of corticotropin-releasing hormone (CRH) and proopiomelanocortin (POMC) genes in human skin. FASEB J 2001; 15(12): 2297-9.
[PMID: 11511529]

[36] Schmid-Ott G, Jaeger B, Boehm T, *et al.* Immunological effects of stress in psoriasis. Br J Dermatol 2009; 160(4): 782-5.
[http://dx.doi.org/10.1111/j.1365-2133.2008.09013.x] [PMID: 19210504]

[37] Bjerke JR, Krogh HK, Matre R. Characterization of mononuclear cell infiltrates in psoriatic lesions. J Invest Dermatol 1978; 71(5): 340-3.
[http://dx.doi.org/10.1111/1523-1747.ep12529841] [PMID: 309493]

[38] Buske-Kirschbaum A, Kern S, Ebrecht M, Hellhammer DH. Altered distribution of leukocyte subsets and cytokine production in response to acute psychosocial stress in patients with psoriasis vulgaris. Brain Behav Immun 2007; 21(1): 92-9.
[http://dx.doi.org/10.1016/j.bbi.2006.03.006] [PMID: 16714097]

[39] Bos JD, De Rie MA. The pathogenesis of psoriasis: immunological facts and speculations. Immunol Today 1999; 20(1): 40-6.
[http://dx.doi.org/10.1016/S0167-5699(98)01381-4] [PMID: 10081229]

[40] Basińska MA, Woźniewicz A. The relation between type D personality and the clinical condition of patients suffering from psoriasis. Postepy Dermatol Alergol 2013; 30(6): 381-7.
[http://dx.doi.org/10.5114/pdia.2013.39437] [PMID: 24494001]

[41] Zeljko-Penavić J, Situm M, Babić D, Simić D. Analysis of psychopathological traits in psoriatic patients. Psychiatr Danub 2013; 25 (Suppl. 1): 56-9.
[PMID: 23806969]

[42] Litaiem N, Youssef S, Jabeur K, Dhaoui MR, Doss N. Affective temperament profile in psoriasis patients in Tunisia using TEMPS-A. J Affect Disord 2013; 151(1): 321-4.
[http://dx.doi.org/10.1016/j.jad.2013.05.099] [PMID: 23830858]

[43] Remröd C, Sjöström K, Svensson A. Psychological differences between early- and late-onset psoriasis:

a study of personality traits, anxiety and depression in psoriasis. Br J Dermatol 2013; 169(2): 344-50. [http://dx.doi.org/10.1111/bjd.12371] [PMID: 23565588]

[44] Magin P, Adams J, Heading G, Pond D, Smith W. The psychological sequelae of psoriasis: results of a qualitative study. Psychol Health Med 2009; 14(2): 150-61. [http://dx.doi.org/10.1080/13548500802512294] [PMID: 19235074]

[45] Remröd C, Sjöström K, Svensson Å. Pruritus in psoriasis: a study of personality traits, depression and anxiety. Acta Derm Venereol 2015; 95(4): 439-43. [http://dx.doi.org/10.2340/00015555-1975] [PMID: 25229695]

[46] Janowski K, Steuden S, Bogaczewicz J. Clinical and psychological characteristics of patients with psoriasis reporting various frequencies of pruritus. Int J Dermatol 2014; 53(7): 820-9. [http://dx.doi.org/10.1111/ijd.12074] [PMID: 24261840]

[47] Heller MM, Wong JW, Nguyen TV, *et al.* Quality-of-life instruments: evaluation of the impact of psoriasis on patients. Dermatol Clin 2012; 30(2): 281-291, ix. [http://dx.doi.org/10.1016/j.det.2011.11.006] [PMID: 22284142]

[48] Koo J. Population-based epidemiologic study of psoriasis with emphasis on quality of life assessment. Dermatol Clin 1996; 14(3): 485-96. [http://dx.doi.org/10.1016/S0733-8635(05)70376-4] [PMID: 8818558]

[49] Gupta MA, Gupta AK, Kirkby S, *et al.* Pruritus in psoriasis. A prospective study of some psychiatric and dermatologic correlates. Arch Dermatol 1988; 124(7): 1052-7. [http://dx.doi.org/10.1001/archderm.1988.01670070040016] [PMID: 3389849]

[50] Yosipovitch G, Goon A, Wee J, Chan YH, Goh CL. The prevalence and clinical characteristics of pruritus among patients with extensive psoriasis. Br J Dermatol 2000; 143(5): 969-73. [http://dx.doi.org/10.1046/j.1365-2133.2000.03829.x] [PMID: 11069504]

[51] Szepietowski JC, Reich A, Wisnicka B. Pruritus and psoriasis. Br J Dermatol 2004; 151(6): 1284. [http://dx.doi.org/10.1111/j.1365-2133.2004.06299.x] [PMID: 15606540]

[52] Reich A, Szepietowski JC. Clinical Aspects of Itch: Psoriasis. In: Carstens E, Akiyama T, Eds. Itch: Mechanisms and Treatment. Boca Raton, FL: CRC press 2014. Chapter 4 [http://dx.doi.org/10.1201/b16573-5]

[53] Reich A, Welz-Kubiak K, Szepietowski JC. Pruritus differences between psoriasis and lichen planus. Acta Derm Venereol 2011; 91(5): 605-6. [http://dx.doi.org/10.2340/00015555-1129] [PMID: 21547340]

[54] Gupta MA, Gupta AK, Schork NJ, Ellis CN. Depression modulates pruritus perception: a study of pruritus in psoriasis, atopic dermatitis, and chronic idiopathic urticaria. Psychosom Med 1994; 56(1): 36-40. [http://dx.doi.org/10.1097/00006842-199401000-00005] [PMID: 8197313]

[55] Zimolag I, Reich A, Szepietowski JC. Influence of psoriasis on the ability to work. Acta Derm Venereol 2009; 89: 575-6.

[56] Zamirska A, Reich A, Berny-Moreno J, Salomon J, Szepietowski JC. Vulvar pruritus and burning sensation in women with psoriasis. Acta Derm Venereol 2008; 88(2): 132-5. [http://dx.doi.org/10.2340/00015555-0372] [PMID: 18311439]

[57] McHenry PM, Doherty VR. Psoriasis: an audit of patients' views on the disease and its treatment. Br J Dermatol 1992; 127(1): 13-7.
[http://dx.doi.org/10.1111/j.1365-2133.1992.tb14817.x] [PMID: 1637688]

[58] Singh P, Soyer HP, Wu J, Salmhofer W, Gilmore S. Tele-assessment of Psoriasis Area and Severity Index: a study of the accuracy of digital image capture. Australas J Dermatol 2011; 52(4): 259-63.
[http://dx.doi.org/10.1111/j.1440-0960.2011.00800.x] [PMID: 22070699]

[59] Fortune DG, Richards HL, Main CJ, Griffiths CE. What patients with psoriasis believe about their condition. J Am Acad Dermatol 1998; 39(2 Pt 1): 196-201.
[http://dx.doi.org/10.1016/S0190-9622(98)70074-X] [PMID: 9704828]

[60] Wahl AK, Gjengedal E, Hanestad BR. The bodily suffering of living with severe psoriasis: in-depth interviews with 22 hospitalized patients with psoriasis. Qual Health Res 2002; 12(2): 250-61.
[http://dx.doi.org/10.1177/104973202129119874] [PMID: 11837374]

[61] Krueger G, Koo J, Lebwohl M, Menter A, Stern RS, Rolstad T. The impact of psoriasis on quality of life: results of a 1998 National Psoriasis Foundation patient-membership survey. Arch Dermatol 2001; 137(3): 280-4.
[PMID: 11255325]

[62] Krueger GG, Feldman SR, Camisa C, *et al.* Two considerations for patients with psoriasis and their clinicians: what defines mild, moderate, and severe psoriasis? What constitutes a clinically significant improvement when treating psoriasis? J Am Acad Dermatol 2000; 43(2 Pt 1): 281-5.
[http://dx.doi.org/10.1067/mjd.2000.106374] [PMID: 10906652]

[63] Pettey AA, Balkrishnan R, Rapp SR, Fleischer AB, Feldman SR. Patients with palmoplantar psoriasis have more physical disability and discomfort than patients with other forms of psoriasis: implications for clinical practice. J Am Acad Dermatol 2003; 49(2): 271-5.
[http://dx.doi.org/10.1067/S0190-9622(03)01479-8] [PMID: 12894076]

[64] Kyriakou A, Patsatsi A, Sotiriadis D. Quality of life and severity of skin and nail involvement in patients with plaque psoriasis. Eur J Dermatol 2014; 24(5): 623-5.
[PMID: 25075721]

[65] Sampogna F, Tabolli S, Söderfeldt B, Axtelius B, Aparo U, Abeni D. IDI Multipurpose Psoriasis Research on Vital Experiences (IMPROVE) investigators. Measuring quality of life of patients with different clinical types of psoriasis using the SF-36. Br J Dermatol 2006; 154(5): 844-9.
[http://dx.doi.org/10.1111/j.1365-2133.2005.07071.x] [PMID: 16634884]

[66] Zachariae H, Zachariae R, Blomqvist K, *et al.* Quality of life and prevalence of arthritis reported by 5795 members of the Nordic Psoriasis Associations: data from the Nordic Quality of Life Study. Acta Derm Venereol 2002; 82(2): 108-13.
[http://dx.doi.org/10.1080/00015550252948130] [PMID: 12125937]

[67] Lundberg L, Johannesson M, Silverdahl M, Hermansson C, Lindberg M. Health-related quality of life in patients with psoriasis and atopic dermatitis measured with SF-36, DLQI and a subjective measure of disease activity. Acta Derm Venereol 2000; 80(6): 430-4.
[http://dx.doi.org/10.1080/000155500300012873] [PMID: 11243637]

[68] Fortune DG, Main CJ, O'Sullivan TM, Griffiths CE. Quality of life in patients with psoriasis: the

contribution of clinical variables and psoriasis-specific stress. Br J Dermatol 1997; 137(5): 755-60. [http://dx.doi.org/10.1111/j.1365-2133.1997.tb01113.x] [PMID: 9415236]

[69] de Korte J, Sprangers MA, Mombers FM, Bos JD. Quality of life in patients with psoriasis: a systematic literature review. J Investig Dermatol Symp Proc 2004; 9(2): 140-7. [http://dx.doi.org/10.1046/j.1087-0024.2003.09110.x] [PMID: 15083781]

[70] Shutty BG, West C, Huang KE, *et al.* Sleep disturbances in psoriasis Dermatol Online J 2013; 19(1): 1.

[71] Stinco G, Trevisan G, Piccirillo F, *et al.* Psoriasis vulgaris does not adversely influence the quality of sleep. G Ital Dermatol Venereol 2013; 148(6): 655-9. [PMID: 24442047]

[72] Leibovici V, Canetti L, Yahalomi S, *et al.* Well being, psychopathology and coping strategies in psoriasis compared with atopic dermatitis: a controlled study. J Eur Acad Dermatol Venereol 2010; 24(8): 897-903. [http://dx.doi.org/10.1111/j.1468-3083.2009.03542.x] [PMID: 20070455]

[73] Vardy D, Besser A, Amir M, Gesthalter B, Biton A, Buskila D. Experiences of stigmatization play a role in mediating the impact of disease severity on quality of life in psoriasis patients. Br J Dermatol 2002; 147(4): 736-42. [http://dx.doi.org/10.1046/j.1365-2133.2002.04899.x] [PMID: 12366421]

[74] Böhm D, Stock Gissendanner S, Bangemann K, *et al.* Perceived relationships between severity of psoriasis symptoms, gender, stigmatization and quality of life. J Eur Acad Dermatol Venereol 2013; 27(2): 220-6. [http://dx.doi.org/10.1111/j.1468-3083.2012.04451.x] [PMID: 22329829]

[75] Hrehorów E, Salomon J, Matusiak L, Reich A, Szepietowski JC. Patients with psoriasis feel stigmatized. Acta Derm Venereol 2012; 92(1): 67-72. [http://dx.doi.org/10.2340/00015555-1193] [PMID: 21879243]

[76] Scharloo M, Kaptein AA, Weinman J, Bergman W, Vermeer BJ, Rooijmans HG. Patients' illness perceptions and coping as predictors of functional status in psoriasis: a 1-year follow-up. Br J Dermatol 2000; 142(5): 899-907. [http://dx.doi.org/10.1046/j.1365-2133.2000.03469.x] [PMID: 10809846]

[77] Herron MD, Hinckley M, Hoffman MS, *et al.* Impact of obesity and smoking on psoriasis presentation and management. Arch Dermatol 2005; 141(12): 1527-34. [http://dx.doi.org/10.1001/archderm.141.12.1527] [PMID: 16365253]

[78] Sathyanarayana Rao TS, Basavaraj KH, Das K. Psychosomatic paradigms in psoriasis: Psoriasis, stress and mental health. Indian J Psychiatry 2013; 55(4): 313-5. [http://dx.doi.org/10.4103/0019-5545.120531] [PMID: 24459298]

[79] Wahl A, Hanestad BR, Wiklund I, Moum T. Coping and quality of life in patients with psoriasis. Qual Life Res 1999; 8(5): 427-33. [http://dx.doi.org/10.1023/A:1008944108101] [PMID: 10474284]

[80] Zalewska A, Miniszewska J, Chodkiewicz J, Narbutt J. Acceptance of chronic illness in psoriasis vulgaris patients. J Eur Acad Dermatol Venereol 2007; 21(2): 235-42.

[http://dx.doi.org/10.1111/j.1468-3083.2006.01912.x] [PMID: 17243960]

[81] Ginsburg IH, Link BG. Psychosocial consequences of rejection and stigma feelings in psoriasis patients. Int J Dermatol 1993; 32(8): 587-91. [http://dx.doi.org/10.1111/j.1365-4362.1993.tb05031.x] [PMID: 8407075]

[82] Pereira MG, Brito L, Smith T. Dyadic adjustment, family coping, body image, quality of life and psychological morbidity in patients with psoriasis and their partners. Int J Behav Med 2012; 19(3): 260-9. [http://dx.doi.org/10.1007/s12529-011-9174-5] [PMID: 21706200]

[83] Eghlileb AM, Davies EE, Finlay AY. Psoriasis has a major secondary impact on the lives of family members and partners. Br J Dermatol 2007; 156(6): 1245-50. [http://dx.doi.org/10.1111/j.1365-2133.2007.07881.x] [PMID: 17459044]

[84] Hawro T, Zalewska A, Hawro M, Kaszuba A, Królikowska M, Maurer M. Impact of psoriasis severity on family income and quality of life. J Eur Acad Dermatol Venereol 2015; 29(3): 438-43. [http://dx.doi.org/10.1111/jdv.12572] [PMID: 24852054]

[85] Weiss SC, Kimball AB, Liewehr DJ, Blauvelt A, Turner ML, Emanuel EJ. Quantifying the harmful effect of psoriasis on health-related quality of life. J Am Acad Dermatol 2002; 47(4): 512-8. [http://dx.doi.org/10.1067/mjd.2002.122755] [PMID: 12271293]

[86] Feldman SR, Fleischer AB Jr, Reboussin DM, *et al.* The economic impact of psoriasis increases with psoriasis severity. J Am Acad Dermatol 1997; 37(4): 564-9. [http://dx.doi.org/10.1016/S0190-9622(97)70172-5] [PMID: 9344194]

[87] Gupta MA, Gupta AK. Age and gender differences in the impact of psoriasis on quality of life. Int J Dermatol 1995; 34(10): 700-3. [http://dx.doi.org/10.1111/j.1365-4362.1995.tb04656.x] [PMID: 8537157]

[88] Linder D, Dall'olio E, Gisondi P, *et al.* Perception of disease and doctor-patient relationship experienced by patients with psoriasis: a questionnaire-based study. Am J Clin Dermatol 2009; 10(5): 325-30. [http://dx.doi.org/10.2165/11311190-000000000-00000] [PMID: 19658445]

[89] American Psychiatric Association. Diagnostic and statistical manual of mental disorders. 5th ed. Washington: American Psychiatric Publishing 2013; pp. 189-95.

[90] Hammerlid E, Ahlner-Elmqvist M, Bjordal K, *et al.* A prospective multicentre study in Sweden and Norway of mental distress and psychiatric morbidity in head and neck cancer patients. Br J Cancer 1999; 80(5-6): 766-74. [http://dx.doi.org/10.1038/sj.bjc.6690420] [PMID: 10360654]

[91] Stangier U, Ehlers A, Gieler U. Measuring adjustment to chronic skin disorders: validation of a self-report measure. Psychol Assess 2003; 15(4): 532-49. [http://dx.doi.org/10.1037/1040-3590.15.4.532] [PMID: 14692848]

[92] [Hayes J, Koo J. Psoriasis: depression, anxiety, smoking, and drinking habits. Dermatol Ther (Heidelb) 2010; 23: 174-80.

[93] Schneider G, Heuft G, Hockmann J. Determinants of social anxiety and social avoidance in psoriasis outpatients. J Eur Acad Dermatol Venereol 2013; 27(3): 383-6.

[http://dx.doi.org/10.1111/j.1468-3083.2011.04307.x] [PMID: 21999164]

[94] Freire M, Rodríguez J, Möller I, *et al.* [Prevalence of symptoms of anxiety and depression in patients with psoriatic arthritis attending rheumatology clinics]. Reumatol Clin 2011; 7(1): 20-6. [Spanish]. [http://dx.doi.org/10.1016/j.reuma.2010.03.003] [PMID: 21794775]

[95] McDonough E, Ayearst R, Eder L, *et al.* Depression and anxiety in psoriatic disease: prevalence and associated factors. J Rheumatol 2014; 41(5): 887-96. [http://dx.doi.org/10.3899/jrheum.130797] [PMID: 24692521]

[96] Pujol RM, Puig L, Daudén E, *et al.* Mental health self-assessment in patients with moderate to severe psoriasis: an observational, multicenter study of 1164 patients in Spain (the VACAP Study). Actas Dermosifiliogr 2013; 104(10): 897-903. [http://dx.doi.org/10.1016/j.adengl.2013.04.019] [PMID: 24112536]

[97] Rieder E, Tausk F. Psoriasis, a model of dermatologic psychosomatic disease: psychiatric implications and treatments. Int J Dermatol 2012; 51(1): 12-26. [http://dx.doi.org/10.1111/j.1365-4632.2011.05071.x] [PMID: 22182372]

[98] Richards HL, Fortune DG, Griffiths CE, Main CJ. The contribution of perceptions of stigmatisation to disability in patients with psoriasis. J Psychosom Res 2001; 50(1): 11-5. [http://dx.doi.org/10.1016/S0022-3999(00)00210-5] [PMID: 11259795]

[99] Consoli SM, Rolhion S, Martin C, *et al.* Low levels of emotional awareness predict a better response to dermatological treatment in patients with psoriasis. Dermatology (Basel) 2006; 212(2): 128-36. [http://dx.doi.org/10.1159/000090653] [PMID: 16484819]

[100] Taner E, Coşar B, Burhanoğlu S, Calikoğlu E, Onder M, Arikan Z. Depression and anxiety in patients with Behçet's disease compared with that in patients with psoriasis. Int J Dermatol 2007; 46(11): 1118-24. [http://dx.doi.org/10.1111/j.1365-4632.2007.03247.x] [PMID: 17988328]

[101] Devrimci-Ozguven H, Kundakci TN, Kumbasar H, Boyvat A. The depression, anxiety, life satisfaction and affective expression levels in psoriasis patients. J Eur Acad Dermatol Venereol 2000; 14(4): 267-71. [http://dx.doi.org/10.1046/j.1468-3083.2000.00085.x] [PMID: 11204514]

[102] Kiliç A, Güleç MY, Gül U, Güleç H. Temperament and character profile of patients with psoriasis. J Eur Acad Dermatol Venereol 2008; 22(5): 537-42. [http://dx.doi.org/10.1111/j.1468-3083.2007.02460.x] [PMID: 18331306]

[103] Kurd SK, Troxel AB, Crits-Christoph P, Gelfand JM. The risk of depression, anxiety, and suicidality in patients with psoriasis: a population-based cohort study. Arch Dermatol 2010; 146(8): 891-5. [PMID: 20713823]

[104] Schmitt J, Ford DE. Understanding the relationship between objective disease severity, psoriatic symptoms, illness-related stress, health-related quality of life and depressive symptoms in patients with psoriasis - a structural equations modeling approach. Gen Hosp Psychiatry 2007; 29(2): 134-40. [http://dx.doi.org/10.1016/j.genhosppsych.2006.12.004] [PMID: 17336662]

[105] Khraishi M, MacDonald D, Rampakakis E, Vaillancourt J, Sampalis JS. Prevalence of patient-reported comorbidities in early and established psoriatic arthritis cohorts. Clin Rheumatol 2011; 30(7): 877-85.

[http://dx.doi.org/10.1007/s10067-011-1692-7] [PMID: 21287359]

[106] Husted JA, Thavaneswaran A, Chandran V, *et al.* Cardiovascular and other comorbidities in patients with psoriatic arthritis: a comparison with patients with psoriasis. Arthritis Care Res (Hoboken) 2011; 63(12): 1729-35.
[http://dx.doi.org/10.1002/acr.20627] [PMID: 21905258]

[107] Kotrulja L, Tadinac M, Joki-Begi NA, Gregurek R. A multivariate analysis of clinical severity, psychological distress and psychopathological traits in psoriatic patients. Acta Derm Venereol 2010; 90(3): 251-6.
[http://dx.doi.org/10.2340/00015555-0838] [PMID: 20526541]

[108] Saraceno R, Faleri S, Ruzzetti M, Centonze D, Chimenti S. Prevalence and management of panic attacks during infliximab infusion in psoriatic patients. Dermatology (Basel) 2012; 225(3): 236-41.
[http://dx.doi.org/10.1159/000343609] [PMID: 23183380]

[109] Daudén E, Griffiths CE, Ortonne JP, *et al.* Improvements in patient-reported outcomes in moderate-t--severe psoriasis patients receiving continuous or paused etanercept treatment over 54 weeks: the CRYSTEL study. J Eur Acad Dermatol Venereol 2009; 23(12): 1374-82.
[http://dx.doi.org/10.1111/j.1468-3083.2009.03321.x] [PMID: 19563497]

[110] Menter A, Augustin M, Signorovitch J, *et al.* The effect of adalimumab on reducing depression symptoms in patients with moderate to severe psoriasis: a randomized clinical trial. J Am Acad Dermatol 2010; 62(5): 812-8.
[http://dx.doi.org/10.1016/j.jaad.2009.07.022] [PMID: 20219265]

[111] Langley RG, Feldman SR, Han C, *et al.* Ustekinumab significantly improves symptoms of anxiety, depression, and skin-related quality of life in patients with moderate-to-severe psoriasis: Results from a randomized, double-blind, placebo-controlled phase III trial. J Am Acad Dermatol 2010; 63(3): 457-65.
[http://dx.doi.org/10.1016/j.jaad.2009.09.014] [PMID: 20462664]

[112] American Psychiatric Association. Diagnostic and statistical manual of mental disorders. 5th ed. Washington: American Psychiatric Publishing 2013; pp. 155-60.

[113] Gupta MA, Gupta AK. Depression and suicidal ideation in dermatology patients with acne, alopecia areata, atopic dermatitis and psoriasis. Br J Dermatol 1998; 139(5): 846-50.
[http://dx.doi.org/10.1046/j.1365-2133.1998.02511.x] [PMID: 9892952]

[114] Akay A, Pekcanlar A, Bozdag KE, Altintas L, Karaman A. Assessment of depression in subjects with psoriasis vulgaris and lichen planus. J Eur Acad Dermatol Venereol 2002; 16(4): 347-52.
[http://dx.doi.org/10.1046/j.1468-3083.2002.00467.x] [PMID: 12224690]

[115] Dowlatshahi E A, Wakkee M, Arends L R, *et al.* The prevalence and odds of depressive symptoms and clinical depression in psoriasis patients: A systematic review and meta-analysis 2014; 134(6): 1542-51.

[116] Picardi A, Mazzotti E, Pasquini P. Prevalence and correlates of suicidal ideation among patients with skin disease. J Am Acad Dermatol 2006; 54(3): 420-6.
[http://dx.doi.org/10.1016/j.jaad.2005.11.1103] [PMID: 16488292]

[117] Gupta MA, Gupta AK, Watteel GN. Perceived deprivation of social touch in psoriasis is associated with greater psychologic morbidity: an index of the stigma experience in dermatologic disorders. Cutis

1998; 61(6): 339-42.
[PMID: 9640555]

[118] Sampogna F, Tabolli S, Mastroeni S, Di Pietro C, Fortes C, Abeni D. Italian Multipurpose Psoriasis Research on Vital Experiences (IMPROVE) study group. Quality of life impairment and psychological distress in elderly patients with psoriasis. Dermatology (Basel) 2007; 215(4): 341-7.
[http://dx.doi.org/10.1159/000107628] [PMID: 17911993]

[119] Miller AH, Maletic V, Raison CL. Inflammation and its discontents: the role of cytokines in the pathophysiology of major depression. Biol Psychiatry 2009; 65(9): 732-41.
[http://dx.doi.org/10.1016/j.biopsych.2008.11.029] [PMID: 19150053]

[120] Schön MP, Boehncke WH. Psoriasis. N Engl J Med 2005; 352(18): 1899-912.
[http://dx.doi.org/10.1056/NEJMra041320] [PMID: 15872205]

[121] Bandinelli F, Prignano F, Bonciani D, *et al.* Clinical and demographic factors influence on anxiety and depression in early psoriatic arthritis (ePsA). Clin Exp Rheumatol 2013; 31(2): 318-9.
[PMID: 23295140]

[122] Biljan D, Laufer D, Filaković P, Situm M, Brataljenović T. Psoriasis, mental disorders and stress. Coll Antropol 2009; 33(3): 889-92.
[PMID: 19860120]

[123] Schmitt JM, Ford DE. Role of depression in quality of life for patients with psoriasis. Dermatology (Basel) 2007; 215(1): 17-27.
[http://dx.doi.org/10.1159/000102029] [PMID: 17587835]

[124] Esposito M, Saraceno R, Giunta A, Maccarone M, Chimenti S. An Italian study on psoriasis and depression. Dermatology (Basel) 2006; 212(2): 123-7.
[http://dx.doi.org/10.1159/000090652] [PMID: 16484818]

[125] Mercan S, Altunay IK, Demir B, Akpinar A, Kayaoglu S. Sexual dysfunctions in patients with neurodermatitis and psoriasis. J Sex Marital Ther 2008; 34(2): 160-8.
[http://dx.doi.org/10.1080/00926230701267951] [PMID: 18224550]

[126] Sampogna F, Gisondi P, Tabolli S, *et al.* IDI Multipurpose Psoriasis Research ON Vital Experiences Investigators. Impairment of sexual life in patients with psoriasis. Dermatology 1997; 36(4): 259-62.

[127] Gupta MA, Gupta AK. Psoriasis and sex: a study of moderately to severely affected patients. Int J Dermatol 1997; 36(4): 259-62.
[http://dx.doi.org/10.1046/j.1365-4362.1997.00032.x] [PMID: 9169321]

[128] Türel Ermertcan A, Temeltaş G, Deveci A, Dinç G, Güler HB, Oztürkcan S. Sexual dysfunction in patients with psoriasis. J Dermatol 2006; 33(11): 772-8.
[http://dx.doi.org/10.1111/j.1346-8138.2006.00179.x] [PMID: 17073992]

[129] Henderson CA, Highet AS. Depression induced by etretinate. BMJ 1989; 298(6678): 964.
[http://dx.doi.org/10.1136/bmj.298.6678.964] [PMID: 2497882]

[130] Ellard R, Ahmed A, Shah R, Bewley A. Suicide and depression in a patient with psoriasis receiving adalimumab: the role of the dermatologist. Clin Exp Dermatol 2014; 39(5): 624-7.
[http://dx.doi.org/10.1111/ced.12351] [PMID: 24934916]

[131] Krishnan R, Cella D, Leonardi C, *et al.* Effects of etanercept therapy on fatigue and symptoms of depression in subjects treated for moderate to severe plaque psoriasis for up to 96 weeks. Br J Dermatol 2007; 157(6): 1275-7.
[http://dx.doi.org/10.1111/j.1365-2133.2007.08205.x] [PMID: 17916204]

[132] Bassukas ID, Hyphantis T, Gamvroulia C, Gaitanis G, Mavreas V. Infliximab for patients with plaque psoriasis and severe psychiatric comorbidity. J Eur Acad Dermatol Venereol 2008; 22(2): 257-8.
[PMID: 18211435]

[133] Ahmed I, Ahmed S, Nasreen S. Frequency and pattern of psychiatric disorders in patients with vitiligo. J Ayub Med Coll Abbottabad 2007; 19(3): 19-21.
[PMID: 18444584]

[134] Sukan M, Maner F. The problems in sexual functions of vitiligo and chronic urticaria patients. J Sex Marital Ther 2007; 33(1): 55-64.
[http://dx.doi.org/10.1080/00926230600998482] [PMID: 17162488]

[135] Al-Mazeedi K, El-Shazly M, Al-Ajmi HS. Impact of psoriasis on quality of life in Kuwait. Int J Dermatol 2006; 45(4): 418-24.
[http://dx.doi.org/10.1111/j.1365-4632.2006.02502.x] [PMID: 16650169]

[136] Meeuwis KA, de Hullu JA, van de Nieuwenhof HP, *et al.* Quality of life and sexual health in patients with genital psoriasis. Br J Dermatol 2011; 164(6): 1247-55.
[http://dx.doi.org/10.1111/j.1365-2133.2011.10249.x] [PMID: 21332459]

[137] Guenther L, Han C, Szapary P, *et al.* Impact of ustekinumab on health-related quality of life and sexual difficulties associated with psoriasis: results from two phase III clinical trials. J Eur Acad Dermatol Venereol 2011; 25(7): 851-7.
[http://dx.doi.org/10.1111/j.1468-3083.2011.04082.x] [PMID: 21521375]

[138] Weinstein MZ. Psychosocial perspectives on psoriasis. Dermatol Clin 1984; 2: 507-15.

[139] Cabete J, Torres T, Vilarinho T, Ferreira A, Selores M. Erectile dysfunction in psoriasis patients. Eur J Dermatol 2014; 24(4): 482-6.
[PMID: 25118566]

[140] Ruiz-Villaverde R, Sánchez-Cano D, Rodrigo JR, Gutierrez CV. Pilot study of sexual dysfunction in patients with psoriasis: influence of biologic therapy. Indian J Dermatol 2011; 56(6): 694-9.
[http://dx.doi.org/10.4103/0019-5154.91831] [PMID: 22345773]

[141] Goulding JM, Price CL, Defty CL, Hulangamuwa CS, Bader E, Ahmed I. Erectile dysfunction in patients with psoriasis: increased prevalence, an unmet need, and a chance to intervene. Br J Dermatol 2011; 164(1): 103-9.
[http://dx.doi.org/10.1111/j.1365-2133.2010.10077.x] [PMID: 20874856]

[142] Kurizky PS, Mota LM. Sexual dysfunction in patients with psoriasis and psoriatic arthritis--a systematic review. Rev Bras Reumatol 2012; 52(6): 943-8.
[http://dx.doi.org/10.1590/S0482-50042012000600011] [PMID: 23223703]

[143] Farber EM, Nall ML. The natural history of psoriasis in 5,600 patients. Dermatologica 1974; 148(1): 1-18.
[http://dx.doi.org/10.1159/000251595] [PMID: 4831963]

[144] Molina-Leyva A, Almodovar-Real A, Ruiz-Carrascosa JC, Naranjo-Sintes R, Serrano-Ortega S, Jimenez-Moleon JJ. Distribution pattern of psoriasis affects sexual function in moderate to severe psoriasis: a prospective case series study. J Sex Med 2014; 11(12): 2882-9.
[http://dx.doi.org/10.1111/jsm.12710] [PMID: 25266400]

[145] Wylie G, Evans CD, Gupta G. Reduced libido and erectile dysfunction: rarely reported side-effects of methotrexate. Clin Exp Dermatol 2009; 34(7): e234.
[http://dx.doi.org/10.1111/j.1365-2230.2008.03082.x] [PMID: 19323665]

[146] Aguirre MA, Vélez A, Romero M, Collantes E. Gynecomastia and sexual impotence associated with methotrexate treatment. J Rheumatol 2002; 29(8): 1793-4.
[PMID: 12180746]

[147] Reynolds OD. Erectile dysfunction in etretinate treatment. Arch Dermatol 1991; 127(3): 425-6.
[http://dx.doi.org/10.1001/archderm.1991.01680030151029] [PMID: 1998382]

[148] Armstrong AW, Harskamp CT, Dhillon JS, Armstrong EJ. Psoriasis and smoking: a systematic review and meta-analysis. Br J Dermatol 2014; 170(2): 304-14.
[http://dx.doi.org/10.1111/bjd.12670] [PMID: 24117435]

[149] Setty AR, Curhan G, Choi HK. Smoking and the risk of psoriasis in women: Nurses' Health Study II. Am J Med 2007; 120(11): 953-9.
[http://dx.doi.org/10.1016/j.amjmed.2007.06.020] [PMID: 17976422]

[150] La Vecchia C, Gallus S, Naldi L. Tobacco and skin disease. Dermatology (Basel) 2005; 211(2): 81-3.
[http://dx.doi.org/10.1159/000086433] [PMID: 16088150]

[151] Horreau C, Pouplard C, Brenaut E, *et al.* Cardiovascular morbidity and mortality in psoriasis and psoriatic arthritis: a systematic literature review. J Eur Acad Dermatol Venereol 2013; 27 (Suppl. 3): 12-29.
[http://dx.doi.org/10.1111/jdv.12163] [PMID: 23845149]

[152] Richard MA, Barnetche T, Horreau C, *et al.* Psoriasis, cardiovascular events, cancer risk and alcohol use: evidence-based recommendations based on systematic review and expert opinion. J Eur Acad Dermatol Venereol 2013; 27 (Suppl. 3): 2-11.
[http://dx.doi.org/10.1111/jdv.12162] [PMID: 23845148]

[153] Pouplard C, Brenaut E, Horreau C, *et al.* Risk of cancer in psoriasis: a systematic review and meta-analysis of epidemiological studies. J Eur Acad Dermatol Venereol 2013; 27 (Suppl. 3): 36-46.
[http://dx.doi.org/10.1111/jdv.12165] [PMID: 23845151]

[154] Farber EM, Nall L. Psoriasis and alcoholism. Cutis 1994; 53(1): 21-7.
[PMID: 8119074]

[155] Wolf R, Wolf D, Ruocco V. Alcohol intake and psoriasis. Clin Dermatol 1999; 17(4): 423-30.
[http://dx.doi.org/10.1016/S0738-081X(99)00028-0] [PMID: 10497727]

[156] Menter A, Griffiths CE, Tebbey PW, Horn EJ, Sterry W. International Psoriasis Council. Exploring the association between cardiovascular and other disease-related risk factors in the psoriasis population: the need for increased understanding across the medical community. J Eur Acad Dermatol Venereol 2010; 24(12): 1371-7.
[http://dx.doi.org/10.1111/j.1468-3083.2010.03656.x] [PMID: 20384692]

[157] Behnam SM, Behnam SE, Koo JY. Alcohol as a risk factor for plaque-type psoriasis. Cutis 2005; 76(3): 181-5.
[PMID: 16268261]

[158] Braathen LR, Botten G, Bjerkedal T. Psoriatics in Norway. A questionnaire study on health status, contact with paramedical professions, and alcohol and tobacco consumption. Acta Derm Venereol Suppl (Stockh) 1989; 142 (Suppl.): 9-12.
[PMID: 2763788]

[159] Lindegård B. Diseases associated with psoriasis in a general population of 159,200 middle-aged, urban, native Swedes. Dermatologica 1986; 172(6): 298-304.
[http://dx.doi.org/10.1159/000249365] [PMID: 3089849]

[160] Fortes C, Mastroeni S, Leffondré K, *et al.* Relationship between smoking and the clinical severity of psoriasis. Arch Dermatol 2005; 141(12): 1580-4.
[http://dx.doi.org/10.1001/archderm.141.12.1580] [PMID: 16365261]

[161] Bø K, Thoresen M, Dalgard F. Smokers report more psoriasis, but not atopic dermatitis or hand eczema: results from a Norwegian population survey among adults. Dermatology (Basel) 2008; 216(1): 40-5.
[http://dx.doi.org/10.1159/000109357] [PMID: 18032898]

[162] Farkas A, Kemény L. Psoriasis and alcohol: is cutaneous ethanol one of the missing links? Br J Dermatol 2010; 162(4): 711-6.
[http://dx.doi.org/10.1111/j.1365-2133.2009.09595.x] [PMID: 19922527]

[163] Brand RM, Jendrzejewski JL, Henery EM, Charron AR. A single oral dose of ethanol can alter transdermal absorption of topically applied chemicals in rats. Toxicol Sci 2006; 92(2): 349-55.
[http://dx.doi.org/10.1093/toxsci/kfl010] [PMID: 16679347]

[164] Sakai JT, Mikulich-Gilbertson SK, Long RJ, Crowley TJ. Validity of transdermal alcohol monitoring: fixed and self-regulated dosing. Alcohol Clin Exp Res 2006; 30(1): 26-33.
[http://dx.doi.org/10.1111/j.1530-0277.2006.00004.x] [PMID: 16433729]

[165] Higgins EM, du Vivier AW. Alcohol abuse and treatment resistance in skin disease. J Am Acad Dermatol 1994; 30(6): 1048. [letter].
[http://dx.doi.org/10.1016/S0190-9622(09)80167-9] [PMID: 8188882]

[166] Higgins EM, du Vivier AW. Cutaneous disease and alcohol misuse. Br Med Bull 1994; 50(1): 85-98.
[PMID: 7908595]

[167] Higgins EM, du Vivier AW. Alcohol and the skin. Alcohol Alcohol 1992; 27(6): 595-602.
[PMID: 1292432]

[168] Adamzik K, McAleer MA, Kirby B. Alcohol and psoriasis: sobering thoughts. Clin Exp Dermatol 2013; 38(8): 819-22.
[http://dx.doi.org/10.1111/ced.12013] [PMID: 24252076]

[169] Kirby B, Richards HL, Mason DL, Fortune DG, Main CJ, Griffiths CE. Alcohol consumption and psychological distress in patients with psoriasis. Br J Dermatol 2008; 158(1): 138-40.
[PMID: 17999698]

[170] Poikolainen K, Karvonen J, Pukkala E. Excess mortality related to alcohol and smoking among hospital-treated patients with psoriasis. Arch Dermatol 1999; 135(12): 1490-3. [http://dx.doi.org/10.1001/archderm.135.12.1490] [PMID: 10606054]

[171] Tsunoda SM, Harris RZ, Christians U, *et al.* Red wine decreases cyclosporine bioavailability. Clin Pharmacol Ther 2001; 70(5): 462-7. [http://dx.doi.org/10.1016/S0009-9236(01)70992-7] [PMID: 11719733]

[172] Paul MD, Parfrey PS, Smart M, Gault H. The effect of ethanol on serum cyclosporine A levels in renal transplant recipients. Am J Kidney Dis 1987; 10(2): 133-5. [http://dx.doi.org/10.1016/S0272-6386(87)80045-8] [PMID: 3300294]

[173] Schmutz JL, Barbaud A, Trechot P. [Treatment with acitretin and alcohol drinking: a high risk combination]. Ann Dermatol Venereol 2001; 128(11): 1269. [PMID: 11908183]

[174] Fortune DG, Richards HL, Kirby B, McElhone K, Main CJ, Griffiths CE. Successful treatment of psoriasis improves psoriasis-specific but not more general aspects of patients' well-being. Br J Dermatol 2004; 151(6): 1219-26. [http://dx.doi.org/10.1111/j.1365-2133.2004.06222.x] [PMID: 15606518]

[175] Fordham B, Griffiths CE, Bundy C. Can stress reduction interventions improve psoriasis? A review. Psychol Health Med 2013; 18(5): 501-14. [http://dx.doi.org/10.1080/13548506.2012.736625] [PMID: 23116223]

[176] Winchell SA, Watts RA. Relaxation therapies in the treatment of psoriasis and possible pathophysiologic mechanisms. J Am Acad Dermatol 1988; 18(1 Pt 1): 101-4. [http://dx.doi.org/10.1016/S0190-9622(88)70015-8] [PMID: 3279078]

[177] Tausk F, Whitmore SE. A pilot study of hypnosis in the treatment of patients with psoriasis. Psychother Psychosom 1999; 68(4): 221-5. [http://dx.doi.org/10.1159/000012336] [PMID: 10396014]

[178] Shenefelt PD. Hypnosis in dermatology. Arch Dermatol 2000; 136(3): 393-9. [http://dx.doi.org/10.1001/archderm.136.3.393] [PMID: 10724204]

[179] Shenefelt PD. Biofeedback, cognitive-behavioral methods, and hypnosis in dermatology: is it all in your mind? Dermatol Ther (Heidelb) 2003; 16(2): 114-22. [http://dx.doi.org/10.1046/j.1529-8019.2003.01620.x] [PMID: 12919113]

[180] Goodman M. An hypothesis explaining the successful treatment of psoriasis with thermal biofeedback: a case report. Biofeedback Self Regul 1994; 19(4): 347-52. [http://dx.doi.org/10.1007/BF01776734] [PMID: 7880910]

[181] Price ML, Mottahedin I, Mayo PR. Can psychotherapy help patients with psoriasis? Clin Exp Dermatol 1991; 16(2): 114-7. [http://dx.doi.org/10.1111/j.1365-2230.1991.tb00319.x] [PMID: 2032371]

[182] Fortune DG, Richards HL, Kirby B, Bowcock S, Main CJ, Griffiths CE. A cognitive-behavioural symptom management programme as an adjunct in psoriasis therapy. Br J Dermatol 2002; 146(3): 458-65. [http://dx.doi.org/10.1046/j.1365-2133.2002.04622.x] [PMID: 11952546]

[183] Fortune DG, Richards HL, Griffiths CE, Main CJ. Targeting cognitive-behaviour therapy to patients' implicit model of psoriasis: results from a patient preference controlled trial. Br J Clin Psychol 2004; 43(Pt 1): 65-82.
[http://dx.doi.org/10.1348/014466504772812977] [PMID: 15005907]

[184] Fordham BA, Nelson P, Griffiths CE, Bundy C. The acceptability and usefulness of mindfulness-based cognitive therapy for people living with psoriasis: a qualitative study. Br J Dermatol 2015; 172(3): 823-5.
[http://dx.doi.org/10.1111/bjd.13333] [PMID: 25112782]

[185] Fordham B, Griffiths CE, Bundy C. A pilot study examining mindfulness-based cognitive therapy in psoriasis. Psychol Health Med 2015; 20(1): 121-7.
[http://dx.doi.org/10.1080/13548506.2014.902483] [PMID: 24684520]

[186] Kabat-Zinn J, Wheeler E, Light T, *et al.* Influence of a mindfulness meditation-based stress reduction intervention on rates of skin clearing in patients with moderate to severe psoriasis undergoing phototherapy (UVB) and photochemotherapy (PUVA). Psychosom Med 1998; 60(5): 625-32. [See comment in PubMed Commons below].
[http://dx.doi.org/10.1097/00006842-199809000-00020] [PMID: 9773769]

[187] Benhard JD, Kristeller J, Kabat-Zinn J. Effectiveness of relaxation and visualization techniques as an adjunct to phototherapy and photochemotherapy of psoriasis. J Am Acad Dermatol 1988; 19(3): 572-4.
[http://dx.doi.org/10.1016/S0190-9622(88)80329-3] [PMID: 3049703]

[188] Bundy C, Pinder B, Bucci S, Reeves D, Griffiths CE, Tarrier N. A novel, web-based, psychological intervention for people with psoriasis: the electronic Targeted Intervention for Psoriasis (eTIPs) study. Br J Dermatol 2013; 169(2): 329-36.
[http://dx.doi.org/10.1111/bjd.12350] [PMID: 23551271]

[189] Basavaraj KH, Navya MA, Rashmi R. Stress and quality of life in psoriasis: an update. Int J Dermatol 2011; 50(7): 783-92.
[http://dx.doi.org/10.1111/j.1365-4632.2010.04844.x] [PMID: 21699511]

[190] Farber EM, Nall L. The office visit and the self-help concept in treating the patient with psoriasis: a strategy revisited. Cutis 1993; 51(4): 236-40.
[PMID: 8477602]

[191] Muftin Z, Thompson AR. A systematic review of self-help for disfigurement: effectiveness, usability, and acceptability. Body Image 2013; 10(4): 442-50.
[http://dx.doi.org/10.1016/j.bodyim.2013.07.005] [PMID: 23962642]

[192] Ulnik J. Skin in psychoanalysis. Karnac Books Ltd. 2007; pp. 72-6.

[193] Gupta MA, Guptat AK. The use of antidepressant drugs in dermatology. J Eur Acad Dermatol Venereol 2001; 15(6): 512-8.
[http://dx.doi.org/10.1046/j.1468-3083.2001.00278.x] [PMID: 11843209]

[194] D'Erme AM, Zanieri F, Campolmi E, *et al.* Therapeutic implications of adding the psychotropic drug escitalopram in the treatment of patients suffering from moderate-severe psoriasis and psychiatric comorbidity: a retrospective study. J Eur Acad Dermatol Venereol 2014; 28(2): 246-9.
[http://dx.doi.org/10.1111/j.1468-3083.2012.04690.x] [PMID: 22963277]

CHAPTER 3

Acne Vulgaris: Psychological State

Lucia Tomas-Aragones[2,3,*] and **Servando E. Marron**[1,3]

[1] *Alcañiz Hospital, Zaragoza, Spain*

[2] *University of Zaragoza, Zaragoza, Spain*

[3] *Aragon Health Sciences Institute (IACS), Zaragoza, Spain*

Abstract: Acne is a multifactorial disorder of the pilosebaceous units. Although many forms of acne can affect all age groups, it is most common in adolescence, when it can be prevalent in up to 80% of the population. Acne vulgaris is often considered a minor disorder, however, it is important to appreciate that the condition can result in severe psychological and social disturbances. Healthcare professionals often underestimate the adverse effects of acne and may lack an empathetic attitude towards the emotional suffering of their patients. It is important to remember that although acne is not a life-threatening disease, it can cause distress and adverse psychosocial consequences such as depression, poor self-esteem, and social phobia. Body dysmorphic disorder and suicide ideation should also be screened for in patients presenting with poor self-esteem and a lack of social interaction. An association between acne and impaired health-related quality of life has also been described. This work aims to highlight the importance of acknowledging the psychological effects of acne and providing patients with effective support. Psychological comorbidities, assessment and treatment options are described.

Keywords: Acne vulgaris, Anxiety, Appearance concern, Biopsychosocial model, Body dysmorphic disorder, Body image, Comorbidity, Coping, Emotional distress, Excoriation disorder, Obsessive-compulsive disorder, Psychological assessment, Psychosocial factors, Psychological intervention, Quality of life, Self-esteem, Self-confidence, Social phobia, Stress, Suicide ideation.

* **Corresponding author Lucia Tomas-Aragones:** Alcañiz Hospital and University of Zaragoza, Aragon Health Sciences Institute (IACS), Zaragoza, Spain; Tel. +34 606 973 09; E-mail:ltomas@unizar.es

Klas Nordlind & Anna Zalewska-Janowska (Eds.)

INTRODUCTION

Although acne is often considered a minor disorder, it is important to appreciate that the condition can result in severe psychological and social disturbances. However, healthcare professionals often underestimate the adverse effects of acne. This work aims to highlight the importance of acknowledging the psychological effects of acne and providing patients with effective support.

Acne

Acne is a multifactorial disorder of the pilosebaceous units. Although many forms of acne can affect all age groups, it is most common in adolescence, when it can be prevalent in up to 80% of the population [1].

Acne vulgaris (Fig. **1**) is one of the most common and visible skin diseases encountered by dermatologists in patients between 15 and 40 years old in the United States [2]. Although acne has usually been considered as an adolescent condition, research and clinical findings from the last two decades have shown that it is also frequent in adult population.

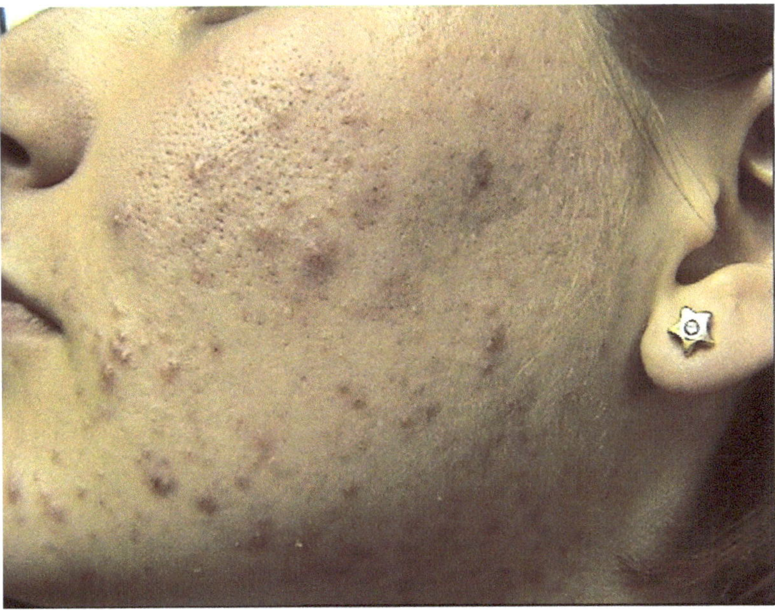

Fig. (1). Moderate acne vulgaris

Acne is not a life-threatening disease, however, it can cause distress and adverse psychosocial consequences such as depression, poor self-esteem, and social phobia. In their research article, Yang *et al.* [3] highlight that acne is an early onset and chronic skin disease, which may influence mental health throughout lifetime, especially in females. Therefore, acne should not be considered simply as a superficial problem in physical appearance. Screening for psychological comorbidities such as major depression and suicide is highly recommended.

Facial acne has been described as a multifactorial disease regarding its pathophysiology and its impact on daily functioning [4, 5]. It has been associated with impaired health related quality of life (HRQoL), and has even been compared with an impact as negative as that of other life-threating diseases [2, 6]. Some studies have shown that facial acne can have a negative impact on self-image, self-confidence and on the ability to establish social relationships [2, 7]. Due to its visibility, acne has a marked psychosocial impact on both adolescents and adults.

We need to remember that the face is the most conspicuous part of our appearance, and together with speech, the most important elements in communication with others. It is therefore clear that acne on the face is going to affect most youngsters negatively [8].

Health professionals are sometimes dismissive of the psychosocial implications of dermatological disorders and lack an empathetic attitude towards the emotional suffering of their patients [9]. The psychosocial impact of acne has been particularly well-documented in adolescents [10, 12]. Health professionals need to bear in mind that patients who suffer from moderate to severe acne, will probably be having difficulties with body image, self-esteem and social interaction [8, 12].

Psychological Impact of Acne

The psychological impact of acne usually consists of a two-way interaction: visible acne lesions may induce negative affects, which may in turn exacerbate the acne. Adolescence is the period of highest risk, not only for acne, but also for mood swings. It is important to bear in mind the difference between psychological disorders that are induced or exacerbated by acne, and the psychiatric comorbidities that are sometimes found in patients with acne, although less clearly linked to the skin condition. Thus, physicians in general and dermatologists in particular, must be careful not to dismiss a "few pimples" [13].

The negative psychological effects of acne can be classified into various categories such as: a) psychological problems related to self-image and self-esteem, as well as feeling embarrassed, angry and frustrated; b) psychosocial problems including self-consciousness during interpersonal relationships related to the feeling of being judged, coping difficulties related to low self-confidence, and low social assertiveness; and c) the resulting behaviour disturbances such as avoidance strategies, use of camouflage makeup, and attempts to control the lesions [13].

The emotional response each patient experiences can be influenced by a variety of factors, such as age, clinical severity of the disease, coping style, family and peer support systems, the psychosocial development of the subject, and other possible underlying psychopathology [8].

Special attention needs to be taken with adolescents, as this age group is especially vulnerable to negative psychological issues. This is partly explained by the hormonally and emotionally volatile period they are experiencing. Therefore, sensitive issues such as body image, dating, social and academic competence, and facing a potentially disfiguring skin condition, can sum up to feelings of self-depreciation, as well as experiences of interpersonal rejection [8].

The Biopsychosocial Model

There is a reciprocal relationship between the skin and the psyche, which is described in the biopsychosocial model that takes into account biological, social and psychological processes in an attempt to provide a more holistic approach to care. The biomedical perspective tends to ignore cognitive or behavioural factors, which may cause or exacerbate a condition. On the other hand, the biopsychosocial model takes into account factors such as social support and psychological stress, as well as factors relating to physiological disorders or the presence of viruses. Mind and body cannot be separated in relation to health since both influence a person's status [14].

Age of Onset

The age of appearance is an important factor regarding looks. Adolescence is when acne occurs most; for example, in the UK up to 95 percent of males and 83 percent of females experience some form of acne before the age of 21 years [15]. According to research, many adolescents suffer emotional distress as a result of their acne [16, 17]. A study carried out by Lasek *et al.* [17] reveals that 70 percent of patients with acne, aged 30-39, reported that their appearance was the most worrisome aspect of their acne compared with 33 percent of those aged 17-19 years. Another interesting finding was that for each decade of life, the negative effects on quality of life increased approximately 20 percent. Older adults were the group most affected by their acne.

Although acne is usually associated with adolescence, acne between 18 and 25 years of age is not less problematic. Late adolescence is a time for making life-shaping decisions, and during this period self-image determines the level of confidence in the transition to adulthood. In a study published by Dalgard *et al.* [18], 3775 individuals aged 18 to 19 years in Norway were assessed for satisfaction with their body and self-esteem. Scores were significantly lower in individuals with acne. More specifically, major impairments were found in self-attitude in males and self-worth in females. Thus, the burden of the visible skin disease is interpreted differently, and the way in which this burden is expressed varies depending on the expectations imposed by society on males and females.

Adults with acne may experience psychological difficulties equal to people with long-term conditions such as diabetes and asthma [19]. Greater employment difficulties have also been reported. Ayer and Burrows [20] informed that as many as 22% of respondents felt that they had been turned down for employment because of their acne.

Appearance Concern

Hassan *et al.* [21] study the effects of gender, age, acne severity and location, on concerns about appearance in people with acne. Almost all the sample (90.1%) showed an important concern about their acne. Once more, this study shows that the older group was more self-consciousness about their appearance. With regards to gender, women showed greater concern than men in concerns related to social, sexual and bodily aspects. On the whole, men had a more positive self-concept than women. The findings of this study demonstrate the impact that acne has on appearance concerns in a group of patients seen at a specialist acne clinic.

According to Pawin *et al.* [22], existential anxiety related to the separation-individuation process is an inherent feature of adolescence. Adolescents often attempt to contain existential anxiety by confining it within their changing body. Thus, acne may serve as an anchor for anxiety, which may become obsessive, leading to self-image impairment that may increase the risk of a depressive disorder.

In their analysis of systematic reviews on acne, Bhate and Williams [23], conclude their findings with some implications for practice, the first one being that acne can have important consequences on both psychological suffering and diminished QoL. It is therefore important to ask patients about these issues.

Sexual Health

Skin conditions, in this case acne, can influence lifestyle choices. For example, a person who feels isolated and unattractive may enter into relationships to feel loved and desired. Because of the link between hormones and acne, female adolescents may also consider oral contraception as a treatment for the condition. This combined with low self-esteem, could increase the possibility of risky sexual behaviour, including an increased risk of pregnancy and sexually transmitted diseases [24].

Stress

Many patients believe stress to be a determining factor in the initiation or aggravation of acne. Stress can increase the levels of glucocorticoids and androgens, which could cause the onset or aggravate acne outbreaks [8]. Although the onset of acne is probably caused by a more complex and multifactorial process, stress could well be a part of this process.

It is important to remember that by influencing negatively on self-esteem, acne may exacerbate the depressive affects considered normal during adolescence. In the event of a stressful event, these negative affects may become stronger and longer lasting, increasing the risk of a depressive disorder. Consequently, body image concerns that seem out of proportion with the objective severity of the lesions may reflect an underlying mood disorder [13].

There are complex, two-sided connections between dermatological conditions and psychological factors, such as atopic dermatitis, psoriasis, alopecia areata, vitiligo and acne [6]. These psychological factors include depression, anxiety, shame, helplessness and anger, and can be grouped under the general term of emotional distress. The symptoms of emotional distress vary in different skin conditions. Parna *et al.* [25], in a study with 176 persons, among which were 40 patients with acne, found that both depression (40%) and general anxiety (39%) symptoms were found in this group of patients. Compared with the control group, patient with acne had considerably more general anxiety ($p=0.006$) [25].

Burden of Acne

In their study, Pawin *et al.* [22], described patients' personal experience of acne, its severity and its treatment. The results show that over half the sample (51%) had not asked for medical attention. However, they said that acne has a significant psychological burden, similar to that of more severe health conditions. The study emphasizes the important psychological impact of acne and highlights the need for young people to be informed that acne can be treated.

Acne is often unaesthetic and can increase an individual's self-consciousness and lead to social stigmatization, resulting in social withdrawal, underachievement at school or work, and even serious psychological problems. We need to remember that the skin is a fundamental organ in communication that plays an important role in socialization throughout one's life cycle [26].

Patients with acne sometimes blame themselves for the condition. They may feel that it is their fault for eating the wrong food [27]. However, evidence of the relationship between diet and acne is generally not clear, although a healthy diet is recommended. Also, some individuals with acne feel that they have caused their acne because of their use of make-up. Once more, although evidence of this is limited, it is recommended that oil-free and non-comedogenic make-up should be used.

Racial Differences

Callender *et al.* [28] studied the racial differences in variables such as clinical characteristics, psychosocial burden, behaviours, perceptions and treatment satisfaction in 208 adult women with facial acne. Age of acne onset and acne concern occurred earlier in white/Caucasian than in non-white/Caucasian subjects. Facial acne affected both groups' quality of life in a negative way, and >70% of the participants described depressive and/or anxiety symptoms [28].

Coping with Acne

Adjustment to a skin condition varies greatly in individuals; some people cope quite well whist others can suffer from depression or anxiety. Interestingly, these differences are not merely the consequence of the severity of the disease; they are the outcome of the interaction of variables that include social skills, social support, perceptions of self-efficacy, optimism and coping style. For example, the impact of stress is a personal, subjective experience that will affect people to varying degrees depending upon their perception of how unpleasant a particular stressor is, and the coping mechanisms that they have to cope with it [14].

Acne can alter body image, and in some cases, cause disfigurement. Given the social significance of one's appearance, many of the problems identified stem from social encounters and reactions from others. The amount of social support a person can draw on, their social skills, levels of optimism and their beliefs about the skin condition all affect the way in which people with specific stressors cope. Evidence from research suggests there is no single mode, which accounts for why some people can adapt well to the challenges of disfigurement while others cannot. However, equipping people with specific coping strategies can definitely alter their capacity to deal with their condition [14].

COMORBIDITIES

Acne is often regarded as a purely cosmetic disorder. However, a review of the literature shows that compared to controls, acne patients show increased levels of anxiety and anger [29, 30], impoverished self-image [31], and an association between the severity of the acne and clinical depression [32]. Furthermore, patients feel their acne to be a source of emotional distress [33], and symptoms such as depression, anxiety, anger, frustration and low self-confidence are quite common in acne patients [12]. Fortunately, these psychological consequences are not permanent and an effective acne treatment can result in the improvement of many of these negative symptoms [33, 34].

Adolescents usually become self-conscious – and sometimes anxious – about their physical changes. They often spend large amounts of time grooming themselves and worrying about how they look. They have a need to be accepted and liked; thus it is quite normal for them to seek recognition from their peers [35].

According to Erikson [36], the quest for identity is the principal developmental task confronting every individual throughout the lifespan – a quest that assumes a different form at each of the various developmental stages the individual passes through. According to Erickson, adolescence is the most severe challenge to young people in their attempt to establish an individual identity. It is then that they are likely to experience an identity crisis that represents a period of confusion and low self-esteem.

It is a crisis because the post-puberty individual is simultaneously confronted by a changed body image, by the new pressures of sexuality, and by the need to make crucial choices, all giving rise to considerable emotional upheaval and making this a time of conflict and uncertainty [37]. It is usually during adolescence that an inner image of oneself is formed, and this is sometimes very different to how others perceive them.

Body image affects our emotions, thoughts, and behaviours in everyday life. But, above all, body image influences our relationships. Furthermore, body image has the potential to dramatically influence our quality of life.

Emotional Distress

Adolescence is a period especially associated with psychological distress. Adolescents often feel vulnerable and sensitive to the changes in their bodies and to their appearance. Research has revealed the burden of acne and its negative effect on patients' quality of life, as well as the impact on self-esteem [7, 8]. Acne-related psychological suffering is associated with mental health disorders such as anxiety, depression, and suicide ideation. It is therefore necessary to screen for psychological and psychiatric disorders in order to be able to offer appropriate treatment.

Anxiety Disorders

Anxiety disorders are often characterized by fear and worry, as well as with associated behavioural disturbances. Anxiety is described as the anticipation of a future threat, while fear is the emotional response to a real or a perceived threat. Although both can overlap, fear is usually associated with the activation of the automatic arousal necessary for flight or flight; there are thoughts of imminent danger and escape behaviours may be necessary. On the other hand, anxiety is normally associated with muscle tension and vigilance; being prepared for danger with avoidant behaviours if necessary. An important number of anxiety disorders develop during childhood and many will persist if not treated [38].

Social Anxiety Disorder (Social Phobia)

Anxiety disorders are characterized by fear of exposing oneself to social situations, and being afraid of feeling scrutinized by others. Individuals with Social Phobia fear that others will judge them in a negative way, for example as weak, stupid, boring, crazy, or unlikeable. These people also feel that they will show anxiety symptoms such as blushing, trembling, sweating or being clumsy, and will be negatively evaluated. As social situations provoke anxiety and fear, individuals who suffer this disorder tend to avoid social interaction [38].

Obsessive-Compulsive Disorder

Individuals with an obsessive-compulsive disorder (OCD) have obsessions and/or compulsions. Obsessions are persistent and recurrent thoughts or urges or images that are often intrusive and unwanted. Compulsions are repetitive behaviours or mental acts that drive the individual with OCD to act according to an obsession or to rules that must be applied in a rigid way. There are other obsessive-compulsive and related disorders that also present with preoccupations and repetitive behaviours or mental acts such as hair pulling, skin picking, *etc*. These recurrent body-focused and repetitive behaviours are also accompanied by repeated attempts to stop the behaviours [38].

Body Dysmorphic Disorder

Body dysmorphic disorder (BDD) is characterized by preoccupations with one or more perceived defects or flaws in one's physical appearance. Individuals with BDD believe they look ugly, unattractive, and abnormal or deformed. These perceived flaws are either slight or not observable to others, yet the bearer can feel hideous, not right or unattractive. Any body area can be the focus of preoccupation and some individuals can have more than one body characteristic they are concerned about. Areas such as the skin, hair, or nose are the most common cause of preoccupation. Perceived asymmetry of body areas is also a preoccupation for some individuals with this disorder. The preoccupations are unwanted, intrusive, difficult to control and time consuming [38].

BDD causes much suffering, is difficult to diagnose and can be a challenge to treat. Patients usually seek treatment for comorbid symptoms of depression, anxiety and social phobia, but few go to a mental health specialist for treatment for BDD symptoms. It is more common for these patients to go to a dermatologist or a plastic surgeon to find a possible solution to their imagined or perceived defect.

Health professionals must be aware that suicidal ideation and even suicide attempts are frequent in patients with BDD. Although further studies are needed to discover the etiology of BDD, effective psychological and psycho-pharmacological treatments are available, hence the importance of asking specific questions about satisfaction with appearance in order to diagnose BDD as early as possible. Early detection in adolescents with BDD is very important as they represent a group of high-risk patients [39].

Screening for BDD in acne patients is therefore a very important task for dermatologists who see these youngsters. The excessive preoccupation with the real or imagined acne lesions is usually associated with impaired psychosocial functioning and possible suicidal thoughts [40].

Excoriation (Skin-Picking) Disorder

Skin-picking or excoriation disorder is characterized by recurrent picking of one's own skin. The face, arms and hands are the most commonly picked sites, however some individuals with this disorder can also pick multiple body sites. Healthy skin, skin with minor irregularities, pimples or calluses, and scabs from previous picking are possible targets to pick. Although some individuals use tweezers, pins or other objects to pick, fingernails are used most frequently to pick the skin. Skin rubbing, squeezing, lancing, and biting are other variations to skin picking. Significant amounts of time are often spent on picking behaviours, some individuals report several hours a day, and this disorder can last for months or even years. Skin picking can cause significant impairment in social, occupational and other areas of functioning, as well as much distress [38].

Scarring is often the result of picking; squeezing and piercing acne lesions can of course worsen the condition. Patients with primary or secondary psychiatric disorders (obsessive-compulsive disorder, mood disorders, body dysmorphic disorder, borderline personality disorder, or delusions of parasitosis) may prove very resistant to treatment because these disorders can predispose them toward picking behaviour [8].

Depressive Disorders

The most common symptoms in depressive disorders are feelings of sadness, emptiness or irritable mood, accompanied by somatic and cognitive changes that significantly affect the capacity to function. The duration, timing and presumed etiology may differ among the different types of depressive disorders: disruptive mood dysregulation disorder, major depressive disorder, dysthymia, premenstrual dysphoric disorder, substance/medication-induced depressive disorder, depressive disorder due to another medical condition, other specified depressive disorder, and unspecified depressive disorder [38].

Marron *et al.* [41], in a study with 346 acne patients, assessed anxiety and depressive symptoms by means of the HADS. During the baseline assessment, 26% were clinical cases for anxiety and 3.5% for depression "The Hospital Anxiety and Depression Scale(HADS)".

Body Image

Social experience and cultural values are largely responsible for a person's perception of his or her attractiveness [42]. Skin blemishes can cause negative reactions from others and this can impact on how an individual experiences and evaluates his or her own attractiveness. On the contrary, smooth and unblemished skin is prized by most western cultures [43, 44]. Women are, on the whole, under greater social pressure to have flawless complexions in comparison to men, and this is more so if the skin condition is in parts of the body that is clearly visible in general encounters [45].

Skin conditions with visible differences, such as acne, can have a negative impact on quality of life [44, 46] where both the social and vocational domains will probably be affected [43].

Healthcare providers should ask acne patients how they feel about their body and themselves in general.

Two simple questions asked during the consultation can screen possible difficulties with body image and can give a lot of valuable information to work further:

On a scale of 1 to 10, how would you rate yourself regarding satisfaction with your appearance?

On a scale of 1 to 10, how would you rate yourself globally, regarding how you feel about yourself in general?

Depending on the answers given, further questions can be asked, such as: What don't you like about your appearance/yourself? How do you think others feel about you? In what way would you like to change? [39].

Suicide Risk

According to the literature, there is evidence of increased suicide risk in patients with psoriasis, atopic dermatitis, and acne, and this risk is higher in patients, whose skin disease is associated with significant emotional distress, alterations in body image, impaired daily activities and difficulties in social interaction. It is therefore important to highlight the important role of the dermatologist in recognizing possible suicidal ideation and being able to help in the prevention of fatal self-harm in their patients [47].

Self-Esteem

Self-esteem is the attitude or worth that the individual has of him or her, and the value given to oneself. A high self-esteem is an important protective factor in coping with being ill, whereas having a poor self-esteem can lead to psychological suffering and mental health disorders [48]. In their study, Dalgard *et al.* [18] describe the association of acne with characteristics such as pride, self-worth, uselessness and body satisfaction among young people (18 year-olds). Their findings reveal that both girls and boys with acne had from depressive symptoms and lower scores in body satisfaction and self-worth than the youngsters in the sample without acne. It is important for dermatologists to remember this when treating young patients with acne.

Quality of Life (QoL)

Acne can profoundly impact quality of life. However, acne severity does not always correlate with the effect on QoL. Effective acne therapy has been associated with significant improvement in quality of life. Dermatologists should consider the disability caused by acne when personalizing a treatment [49].

Marron *et al.* [41], in a study with 346 acne patients, assessed quality of life by means of SF-36 and DLQI. The mean +/- score for DLQI at baseline was 13.2+/-3.7. The Physical Component Summary (PCS) of the SF-36 was 51.7% and the Mental Component Summary (MCS) was 50.8%.

SCREENING FOR PSYCHOLOGICAL COMORBIDITIES AND QUALITY OF LIFE

Getting the patient's perspective is important in clinical practice. For this reason, psychosocial outcome measures have become important in dermatology research as they attempt to examine acne from the perspective of the patient [50].

Approximately 30% of dermatology patients are assessed for psychosocial and psychiatric comorbidity in clinical practice and this provides an important component of the overall evaluation of the patient [51, 52].

Psychometric tools are useful in practice to assess the psychological impact of acne, to detect a possible depressive disorder, to adjust the treatment, and to modulate the interval between scheduled visits, thereby improving treatment adherence and the manner in which the disease is experienced [13].

Quality of Life

General health measures, as well as dermatology-specific measures or acne-specific instruments may be used to measure the impact of acne of quality of life. Measuring quality of life needs to be an easy process in order to incorporate it in the routine clinical work. To make this possible, it is necessary to have instruments that are user-friendly, readily accessible for use and the scores need to be meaningful to the clinician. Health professionals who use theses measures will find that the information obtained can help them to make optimum clinical decisions for their patients, as well as helping them to justify their clinical decisions.

In order to understand the skin condition form the patient's perspective, we need to measure the impact of acne on his/her quality of life. Quality of life questionnaires assess the effect of the condition over the preceding week of the patient's life. Since this can change over time, it is important to repeat the questionnaire at regular intervals to monitor any improvement or deterioration in the patient's QoL. The use of quality of life instruments can result in increased patient satisfaction as the patient gets the message that the healthcare professional is interested in knowing how the skin condition is affecting his/her life. Below, we offer a sample of instruments.

The Dermatology Life Quality Index (DLQI)

[53] is a 10-question dermatology-specific questionnaire that is available in 90 languages. The DLQI is designed for use in adults, over the age of 16. Full information can be found at www.dermatology.org.uk

The Skindex-16

[54] is a 16-question scale to measure how the skin disease affects patients' quality of life. It assesses how affected patients were by their skin problems (*e.g.*, itching, burning, hurting) in the previous week. It encompasses wellbeing in three quality-of-life domains: symptoms, functioning, and emotions.

The Acne-specific quality-of-life questionnaire (Acne-QoL)

[55] is a patient-reported outcome measure that consists of 19 questions to assess the impact of acne (on face) during the last week. It measures four domains: self-perception, role-social, role emotional, and acne symptoms.

The Acne Disability Index (ADI)

[56] assesses the disability caused by acne. This instrument asks about the patients' concern with acne and their degree of self-consciousness. It is a useful questionnaire for identifying patients with poor self-image.

The Cardiff Acne Disability Index (CADI)

[57] is an instrument to be used with teenagers and young adults with acne. It consists of 5 questions. Full information can be found at www.dermatology.org.uk

Psychological Testing

Psychological tests are usually administered and interpreted by a psychologist because of their training in psychopathology and psychometric assessment. Before using a test, it is important to look into its validity and reliability. Feedback on the results should always be offered to the patients.

Body Image

The Derriford Appearance Scale (DAS-59)

[58] consists of 59 items rated on a five-point Likert scale. It is designed to assess the frequency and intensity of affective, cognitive and behavioural issues associated with appearance problems.

The Body Image Disturbance Questionnaire (BIDQ)

[59] measures body image impairment taking into account dissatisfaction, distress and dysfunction. It consists of seven scaled items related to appearance concerns, mental worries with these concerns, and associated experiences of emotional distress, impairment in social and occupation areas, as well as other areas of interference with social life, school, work or role functioning. Behavioural avoidance as a result of the above is also included in the questions of the instrument.

Depression and Anxiety

The Hospital Anxiety and Depression Scale (HADS)

[60], is a 14-item self-report screening scale that was initially used to determine the incidence of anxiety and depression in outpatients with physical illnesses. It consists of two 7-item scales: one for anxiety (HADS-A) and the other for depression (HADS-D) with a range of 0-21.

The Patient Health Questionnaire (PHQ-4)

[61] is a 4-item instrument to measure depressive and anxiety symptoms during the past two weeks. Each item is answered on a 4-point scale with goes from 0 (not at all) to 3 (nearly every day). The total score is interpreted as normal (0-2), mild (3-5), moderate (6-8), or severe (9-12) depression or anxiety.

The Beck Depression Inventory (BDI)

[62] consists of 21 items. It is a self-report inventory that measures symptoms, characteristics and attitudes of depression. The BDI also gives a score on the intensity of depression.

The Center for Epidemiologic Studies Depression Scale (CES-D)

[63] is a 20-question instrument that measures depressive symptoms during the past week in the general population. It uses a scale of 0 – 3.

Self-Esteem

The Rosenberg Self-Esteem Scale (RSES)

[64] evaluates global self-worth with a 10-item self-report questionnaire. It measures both positive and negative feelings about the self.

Others

The Assessment of the Psychological and Social Effects of Acne (ASPEA)

[65] assesses the psychological impact of acne.

The Fear of Negative Evaluation Scale (FNE)

[66] consists of 12 items that measure aspects of social-evaluative anxiety using a scale of 1 to 5. The instrument asks about distress, avoidance and expectations. Being afraid of getting a negative evaluation can be the cause of social anxiety, thus becoming overly concerned with what others think and say of us, and consequently avoiding situations where there is potential evaluation.

TREATMENT

It is important to view the patient in a global and holistic way if we want to understand the psychological suffering related to the skin condition and to be able to offer the best possible treatment. In other words, it is necessary to address the reciprocity between body and mind [14].

The main goals in the treatment of acne are: the prevention of physical sequelae (scars); limitation of the number of intensity of lesions; reduction in the duration of the disease; and minimization of its psychosocial impact [67, 68]. Studies have shown that effective treatment can reduce symptoms of anxiety and depression and significantly improve other physiological parameters [69]. Assessment of psychosocial aspects gives the clinician a better understanding of the patient, and allows them to adjust treatment to the specific needs of each individual.

"High risk" patients are those with functional and psychosocial impairment that may involve self-harm. Being able to recognize these patients in order to offer potent Dermatologic interventions (oral antibiotics or isotretinoin) may help to prevent possible negative outcomes. Others may simply need to be seen on a more regular basis and be given a more empathetic attention in order to achieve a satisfactory outcome. It is necessary to distinguish those patients who require a more intensive psychodermatology intervention from those who would benefit best from psychotropic medication [8].

Oral isotretinoin is a potent retinoid that has been show to be useful in controlling forms of acne that do not respond to the more usual treatment with oral antibiotics and can produce significant physical or emotional scarring [70].

Marron *et al.* [41], in a study with 346 acne patients treated with oral isotretinoin showed a significant improvement in the post-treatment scores of QoL and mood disorders. Their study suggests that oral isotretinoin is not a risk factor for depression and it produces an improvement in symptoms of anxiety and/or depression in patients with mild to moderate acne.

Psychological Intervention

Helping patients to Define their Problem

It is important not to make assumptions about the nature of the patient's problem and the way that it affects him/her. In doing this, there is a danger of over-emphasizing certain issues while ignoring others that may be more pertinent to the patient. In order to avoid making assumptions, the healthcare giver should allow the patient to explain what are the issues that are worrying him/her, and not assume that patients will be able to "open up" and discuss his/her feelings immediately; be patient and let him/her "set the pace". The patient and his/her problem needs to be approached in such a way that it takes into account the complete procure of his/her "illness experience" [14].

What coping strategies are being used?

Patients may have attempted to solve certain problems without success. It is important to know what coping strategies they have used and to find out which did not work and why.

Coping is a dynamic process, which relies on a range of strategies that range from confronting risk and seeking social support to venting emotions and taking comfort in religious beliefs [71].

Strategies for facilitating Change

1. Thought monitoring. Helping patients to become more aware of their thoughts can be achieved by asking them to record when they are feeling emotionally upset and the problem situations in which they find themselves. During the next visit, some of the examples can be discussed and the patient can give alternative rationale responses to the thoughts that have been registered.
2. Thought blocking. This technique is commonly used with people suffering from obsessive disorders. It provides a means of dismissing intrusive thoughts and thus reducing their duration. In the case of acne, recurring thoughts regarding one's appearance are common and patients often find themselves becoming overly anxious regarding how others react to the way that they look and may engage in checking behaviours to see whether the size, number or shape of their lesions has changed. To apply this technique, the patient is asked to describe the different recurring thoughts that they have and when and where these tend to take place. The therapist then asks the patient to describe one of these situations and is asked to put a hand up as soon as he or she begins having the recurring thought. As soon as the patient has raised the hand, the therapist shouts, "Stop"! The patient is asked if the thought has disappeared. This is then repeated with different thoughts and the patient is asked to try "stopping" the thoughts on their own. An alternative to shouting, "stop" is to wear a rubber band around the wrist and to snap it sharply when the recurring thought comes back.
3. Distraction. An effective way of controlling anxiety caused by negative thoughts is through the use of distraction. This technique is useful when patients find themselves becoming anxious. Different tasks can be used, such as: counting how many people are wearing blue shirts or how many people are walking dogs, *etc.* Another task is the use of mental exercises such as reciting the alphabet backwards or counting to one thousand in multiples of 13. Yet

another task would be to recall in detail a pleasant memory or fantasy. Through the use of distraction, anxiety can be controlled and this in turn prevents a vicious cycle from building up whereby negative thoughts create anxiety, which further exacerbates negative thoughts.

4. Graded exposure. The fear and apprehension that a person feels about themselves and others may dominate all aspects of their lives. Patients with acne may cover up their skin with make-up or clothes that conceal the condition, avoid conversations about appearance or avoid activities where there is a possibility of others noticing their condition. One way to help patients cope is by helping them to challenge their beliefs about the feared situation through graded exposure. This involves first establishing with the patient what the feared stimulus is and then constructing a hierarchy of situations that the patient avoids. Only those situations that the patient wishes to overcome are entered on the list. Once the patient has rated the various activities or situations in order of difficulty, they are put into ascending order of least difficult to most difficult and the patient is asked to undertake the least difficult activity on the list. Once the patient has mastered coping with the least anxiety-provoking situation, he or she is asked to move up the list until reaching the most difficult task at the top of the list [14].

Cognitive-Behavioural Therapy

According to cognitive-behavioural therapy (CBT), our perception influences how we think and behave. Therefore, psychological problems are acquired and can be altered through learning processes. Individuals can be taught and helped to identify, challenge and modify problematic thoughts and behaviour patterns that maintain their symptoms.

CBT can be adapted to each person and to his or her problem in particular. With a properly trained health psychologist, CBT can be effective in reducing symptom severity, reducing psychosocial distress and increasing the ability to adjust to the skin condition, and in some cases to control it [72].

Other Interventions

Psychoeducation

Programs providing patients with detailed information about their skin disease, including etiology, therapeutic options, and prognosis, can be helpful in enhancing compliance with treatment regimen. Additionally, psychoeducation directed at educating the patient with regard to common emotional reactions to their skin disease can be helpful in reducing the patient's sense of isolation [73].

Relaxation Training

The association between flare-ups of some skin conditions (*i.e.* psoriasis) and stress has been described [74]. Stress can be the cause of flare-ups, which can lead to more stress. This can then lead to a vicious cycle. Relaxation can prove helpful in reducing arousal levels and consequent feelings of anxiety and stress [72].

Relaxation training can be accomplished by numerous techniques, all mainly orientated at minimizing sympathetic reactivity and enhancing parasympathetic function. Included in this group of procedures are progressive muscle relaxation, autogenic training, guided imagery, as well as transcendental and other meditation techniques, such as mindfulness. Breathing exercises and self-talk have also shown to be helpful [73].

Biofeedback Therapy

Biofeedback, which has wide applications, is a non-invasive conditioning technique. The most commonly used modalities are that of Electromyograph (EMG, muscle tension) and blood flow (temperature) training. In addition to reducing muscle tension and improving blood flow, an overall relaxation response is achieved with this training. Biofeedback training includes a wide variety of progressive muscle-relaxing techniques, imagery techniques, autogenic training, and straightforward conditioning techniques [73].

CONCLUSION

As we have seen, adolescence is characterized both by acne and by mood instability. As a result, teenagers are at high risk for body image impairments and the resulting loss of self-esteem. Healthcare providers should strive to identify patients whose quality-of-life impairments are out of proportion with the severity of the disease. This will help to improve treatment adherence and QoL, to identify patients at high risk for depression and/or suicidal behaviours and, perhaps to minimize social avoidance behaviours in the long term. Efforts to educate teenagers both at school and *via* official websites can mitigate feeling of having to face the disease alone.

CONFLICT OF INTEREST

The authors confirm that they have no conflict of interest to declare for this publication.

ACKNOWLEDGEMENTS

Declared none.

REFERENCES

[1] Rzany B, Kahl C. [Epidemiology of acne vulgaris]. J Dtsch Dermatol Ges 2006; 4(1): 8-9. [http://dx.doi.org/10.1111/j.1610-0387.2005.05876.x] [PMID: 16503926]

[2] Mallon E, Newton JN, Klassen A, Stewart-Brown SL, Ryan TJ, Finlay AY. The quality of life in acne: a comparison with general medical conditions using generic questionnaires. Br J Dermatol 1999; 140(4): 672-6. [http://dx.doi.org/10.1046/j.1365-2133.1999.02768.x] [PMID: 10233319]

[3] Yang Y, Tu H, Hong C, *et al.* Female gender and acne disease are jointly and independently associated with the risk of major depression and suicide: A national population-based study. Biomed Res Int [Internet] 2014. [cited 2014 Nov 12]. ID 504279. Available from: http://www.hindawi.com/journals/bmri/2014/504279/ [http://dx.doi.org/10.1155/2014/504279]

[4] Callender VD. Acne in ethnic skin: special considerations for therapy. Dermatol Ther (Heidelb) 2004; 17(2): 184-95. [http://dx.doi.org/10.1111/j.1396-0296.2004.04019.x] [PMID: 15113286]

[5] Tanghetti EA. Combination therapy is the standard of care. Cutis 2005; 76(2) (Suppl.): 8-14. [PMID: 16164151]

[6] Stern RS. Medication and medical service utilization for acne 1995-1998. J Am Acad Dermatol 2000; 43(6): 1042-8. [http://dx.doi.org/10.1067/mjd.2000.110901] [PMID: 11100021]

[7] Dréno B. Assessing quality of life in patients with acne vulgaris: implications for treatment. Am J Clin Dermatol 2006; 7(2): 99-106.
[http://dx.doi.org/10.2165/00128071-200607020-00003] [PMID: 16605290]

[8] Fried RG, Wechsler A. Psychological problems in the acne patient. Dermatol Ther (Heidelb) 2006; 19(4): 237-40.
[http://dx.doi.org/10.1111/j.1529-8019.2006.00079.x] [PMID: 17004999]

[9] Magin PJ, Adams J, Heading GS, Pond CD. Patients with skin disease and their relationships with their doctors: a qualitative study of patients with acne, psoriasis and eczema. Med J Aust 2009; 190(2): 62-4.
[PMID: 19236289]

[10] Magin P, Adams J, Heading G, Pond D, Smith W. Psychological sequelae of acne vulgaris: results of a qualitative study. Can Fam Physician 2006; 52(8): 978-9.
[PMID: 17273501]

[11] Gupta MA, Gupta AK. Depression and suicidal ideation in dermatology patients with acne, alopecia areata, atopic dermatitis and psoriasis. Br J Dermatol 1998; 139(5): 846-50.
[http://dx.doi.org/10.1046/j.1365-2133.1998.02511.x] [PMID: 9892952]

[12] Koo JY, Smith LL. Psychologic aspects of acne. Pediatr Dermatol 1991; 8(3): 185-8.
[http://dx.doi.org/10.1111/j.1525-1470.1991.tb00856.x] [PMID: 1836060]

[13] Féton-Danou N. [Psychological impact of acne vulgaris]. Ann Dermatol Venereol 2010; 137 (Suppl. 2): S62-5.
[http://dx.doi.org/10.1016/S0151-9638(10)70049-1] [PMID: 21095498]

[14] Papadopoulos L, Bor R, Eds. Psychological approaches to dermatology. Leicester: BPS Books 1999.

[15] Rademaker M, Garioch JJ, Simpson NB. Acne in schoolchildren: no longer a concern for dermatologists. BMJ 1989; 298(6682): 1217-9.
[http://dx.doi.org/10.1136/bmj.298.6682.1217] [PMID: 2526674]

[16] Smithard A, Glazebrook C, Williams HC. Acne prevalence, knowledge about acne and psychological morbidity in mid-adolescence: a community-based study. Br J Dermatol 2001; 145(2): 274-9.
[http://dx.doi.org/10.1046/j.1365-2133.2001.04346.x] [PMID: 11531791]

[17] Lasek RJ, Chren MM. Acne vulgaris and the quality of life of adult dermatology patients. Arch Dermatol 1998; 134(4): 454-8.
[http://dx.doi.org/10.1001/archderm.134.4.454] [PMID: 9554297]

[18] Dalgard F, Gieler U, Holm JO, Bjertness E, Hauser S. Self-esteem and body satisfaction among late adolescents with acne: results from a population survey. J Am Acad Dermatol 2008; 59(5): 746-51.
[http://dx.doi.org/10.1016/j.jaad.2008.07.013] [PMID: 19119094]

[19] Mallon E, Newton JN, Klassen A, Stewart-Brown SL, Ryan TJ, Finlay AY. The quality of life in acne: a comparison with general medical conditions using generic questionnaires. Br J Dermatol 1999; 140(4): 672-6.
[http://dx.doi.org/10.1046/j.1365-2133.1999.02768.x] [PMID: 10233319]

[20] Ayer J, Burrows N. Acne: more than skin deep. Postgrad Med J 2006; 82(970): 500-6.
[http://dx.doi.org/10.1136/pgmj.2006.045377] [PMID: 16891439]

[21] Hassan J, Grogan S, Clark-Carter D, Richards H, Yates VM. The individual health burden of acne: appearance-related distress in male and female adolescents and adults with back, chest and facial acne. J Health Psychol 2009; 14(8): 1105-18.
[http://dx.doi.org/10.1177/1359105309342470] [PMID: 19858331]

[22] Pawin H, Chivot M, Beylot C, *et al.* Living with acne. A study of adolescents' personal experiences. Dermatology (Basel) 2007; 215(4): 308-14.
[http://dx.doi.org/10.1159/000107624] [PMID: 17911988]

[23] Bhate K, Williams HC. What's new in acne? An analysis of systematic reviews published in 2011-2012. Clin Exp Dermatol 2014; 39(3): 273-7.
[http://dx.doi.org/10.1111/ced.12270] [PMID: 24635060]

[24] Bhatti Z, Finlay AY, Salek S. Chronic skin diseases influence major life changing decisions: a new frontier in outcome research. Br J Dermatol 2009; 161 (Suppl. 1): 58-9.

[25] Pärna E, Aluoja A, Kingo K. Quality of life and emotional state in chronic skin disease. Acta Derm Venereol 2015; 95(3): 312-6.
[http://dx.doi.org/10.2340/00015555-1920] [PMID: 24978135]

[26] Panconesi E, Hautmann G. Stress and emotions in skin diseases. In: Koo JY, Lee CS, Eds. Psychocutaneous Medicine. New York: Marcel Dekker 2003; pp. 41-63.

[27] Choices NH. 2014. Available from:http://www.nhs.uk/Conditions/Acne/Pages/Introduction.aspx. [updated 2014 Apr 4; cited 2014 Nov 12].

[28] Callender VD, Alexis AF, Daniels SR, *et al.* Racial differences in clinical characteristics, perceptions and behaviors, and psychosocial impact of adult female acne. J Clin Aesthet Dermatol 2014; 7(7): 19-31.
[PMID: 25053980]

[29] Garrie SA, Garrie EV. Anxiety and skin diseases. Cutis 1978; 22(2): 205-8.
[PMID: 150966]

[30] van der Meeren HL, van der Schaar WW, van den Hurk CM. The psychological impact of severe acne. Cutis 1985; 36(1): 84-6.
[PMID: 3160549]

[31] Shuster S, Fisher GH, Harris E, Binnell D. The effect of skin disease on self image [proceedings]. Br J Dermatol 1978; 99 (Suppl. 16): 18-9.
[http://dx.doi.org/10.1111/j.1365-2133.1978.tb15214.x] [PMID: 151549]

[32] Wu SF, Kinder BN, Trunnell TN, Fulton JE. Role of anxiety and anger in acne patients: a relationship with the severity of the disorder. J Am Acad Dermatol 1988; 18(2 Pt 1): 325-33.
[http://dx.doi.org/10.1016/S0190-9622(88)70047-X] [PMID: 2964458]

[33] Koo J. The psychosocial impact of acne: patients' perceptions. J Am Acad Dermatol 1995; 32(5 Pt 3): S26-30.
[http://dx.doi.org/10.1016/0190-9622(95)90417-4] [PMID: 7738224]

[34] Gupta MA, Gupta AK, Schork NJ, Ellis CN, Voorhees JJ. Psychiatric aspects of the treatment of mild to moderate facial acne. Some preliminary observations. Int J Dermatol 1990; 29(10): 719-21.
[http://dx.doi.org/10.1111/j.1365-4362.1990.tb03777.x] [PMID: 2148562]

[35] Maggit C, Ed. Child development: An illustrated guide. Essex: Heinemann 2006.

[36] Erikson E, Ed. Identity: Youth and crisis. New York: Norton 1968.

[37] Schafer HR, Ed. Key concepts in developmental psychology. London: Sage 2006. [http://dx.doi.org/10.4135/9781446278826]

[38] American Psychiatric Association. Diagnostic and statistical manual of mental disorders (DSM-5). Arlington: American Psychiatric Association 2013.

[39] Tomas-Aragones L, Marron SE. Body dysmorphic disorder in adolescents. In: Tareen RS, Greydanus DE, Jafferany M, Patel DR, Merrick J, Eds. Pediatric psycho-dermatology. Berlin: De Gruyter 2011; pp. 201-15.

[40] Phillips KA. Body dysmorphic disorder: the distress of imagined ugliness. Am J Psychiatry 1991; 148(9): 1138-49. [http://dx.doi.org/10.1176/ajp.148.9.1138] [PMID: 1882990]

[41] Marron SE, Tomas-Aragones L, Boira S. Anxiety, depression, quality of life and patient satisfaction in acne patients treated with oral isotretinoin. Acta Derm Venereol 2013; 93(6): 701-6. [http://dx.doi.org/10.2340/00015555-1638] [PMID: 23727704]

[42] Thomson JK, Heinberg LJ, Altabe M, *et al.* Exacting beauty: Theory Assessment, and treatment of body image disturbance. Washington, DC: American psychological association 1999. [http://dx.doi.org/10.1037/10312-000]

[43] Gupta MA, Johnson AM, Gupta AK. The development of an Acne Quality of Life scale: reliability, validity, and relation to subjective acne severity in mild to moderate acne vulgaris. Acta Derm Venereol 1998; 78(6): 451-6. [http://dx.doi.org/10.1080/000155598442773] [PMID: 9833047]

[44] Loney T, Standage M, Lewis S. Not just 'skin deep': psychosocial effects of dermatological-related social anxiety in a sample of acne patients. J Health Psychol 2008; 13(1): 47-54. [http://dx.doi.org/10.1177/1359105307084311] [PMID: 18086717]

[45] Kellett SC, Gawkrodger DJ. The psychological and emotional impact of acne and the effect of treatment with isotretinoin. Br J Dermatol 1999; 140(2): 273-82. [http://dx.doi.org/10.1046/j.1365-2133.1999.02662.x] [PMID: 10233222]

[46] Cotterill JA, Cunliffe WJ. Suicide in dermatological patients. Br J Dermatol 1997; 137(2): 246-50. [http://dx.doi.org/10.1046/j.1365-2133.1997.18131897.x] [PMID: 9292074]

[47] Picardi A, Lega I, Tarolla E. Suicide risk in skin disorders. Clin Dermatol 2013; 31(1): 47-56. [http://dx.doi.org/10.1016/j.clindermatol.2011.11.006] [PMID: 23245973]

[48] Rosenberg M. Society and the adolescent self-image. Princeton: Princeton University Press 1989.

[49] Zip C. The impact of acne on quality of life. Skin Therapy Lett 2007; 12(10): 7-9. [PMID: 18227954]

[50] Bowe WP, Doyle AK, Crerand CE, Margolis DJ, Shalita AR. Body image disturbance in patients with acne vulgaris. J Clin Aesthet Dermatol 2011; 4(7): 35-41. [PMID: 21779418]

[51] Gupta MA, Gupta AK. Psychodermatology: an update. J Am Acad Dermatol 1996; 34(6): 1030-46. [http://dx.doi.org/10.1016/S0190-9622(96)90284-4] [PMID: 8647969]

[52] Gupta MA, Gupta AK, Ellis CN, Koblenzer CS. Psychiatric evaluation of the dermatology patient. Dermatol Clin 2005; 23(4): 591-9. [http://dx.doi.org/10.1016/j.det.2005.05.005] [PMID: 16112434]

[53] Finlay AY, Khan GK. Dermatology Life Quality Index (DLQI)--a simple practical measure for routine clinical use. Clin Exp Dermatol 1994; 19(3): 210-6. [http://dx.doi.org/10.1111/j.1365-2230.1994.tb01167.x] [PMID: 8033378]

[54] Chren MM, Lasek RJ, Sahay AP, Sands LP. Measurement properties of Skindex-16: a brief quality-o--life measure for patients with skin diseases. J Cutan Med Surg 2001; 5(2): 105-10. [http://dx.doi.org/10.1007/BF02737863] [PMID: 11443481]

[55] Martin AR, Lookingbill DP, Botek A, Light J, Thiboutot D, Girman CJ. Health-related quality of life among patients with facial acne -- assessment of a new acne-specific questionnaire. Clin Exp Dermatol 2001; 26(5): 380-5. [http://dx.doi.org/10.1046/j.1365-2230.2001.00839.x] [PMID: 11488820]

[56] Motley RJ, Finlay AY. How much disability is caused by acne? Clin Exp Dermatol 1989; 14(3): 194-8. [http://dx.doi.org/10.1111/j.1365-2230.1989.tb00930.x] [PMID: 2531637]

[57] Motley RJ, Finlay AY. Practical use of a disability index in the routine management of acne. Clin Exp Dermatol 1992; 17(1): 1-3. [http://dx.doi.org/10.1111/j.1365-2230.1992.tb02521.x] [PMID: 1424249]

[58] Carr AT, Harris DL. The Derriford appearance scale (DAS-59): Instruction on scoring normative data for sub-groups of the general population and the clinical population. Plymouth: University of Plymouth 2000.

[59] Cash T, Phillips K, Santos M, *et al.* Measuring "negative body image": Validation of the body image disturbance questionnaire in a non clinical population. Body Image 2004; 1(4): 363-72. [http://dx.doi.org/10.1016/j.bodyim.2004.10.001]

[60] Zigmond AS, Snaith RP. The hospital anxiety and depression scale. Acta Psychiatr Scand 1983; 67(6): 361-70. [http://dx.doi.org/10.1111/j.1600-0447.1983.tb09716.x] [PMID: 6880820]

[61] Kroenke K, Spitzer RL, Williams JB, Löwe B. An ultra-brief screening scale for anxiety and depression: the PHQ-4. Psychosomatics 2009; 50(6): 613-21. [PMID: 19996233]

[62] Beck AT, Ward CH, Mendelson M, Mock J, Erbaugh J. An inventory for measuring depression. Arch Gen Psychiatry 1961; 4: 561-71. [http://dx.doi.org/10.1001/archpsyc.1961.01710120031004] [PMID: 13688369]

[63] Radloff L. The CES-D Scale: a self-report depression scale for research in the general population. Appl Psychol Meas 1977; 1(3): 381-01. [http://dx.doi.org/10.1177/014662167700100306]

[64] Rosemberg M. Society and the adolescent self image. Princeton: Princeton University Press 1965.

[65] Layton A, Thiboutot D, Bettoli V, Eds. Fast facts: Acne health. Oxford: Health Press Limited 2004.

[66] Leary M. A brief version of the fear of negative evaluation scale. Pers Soc Psychol Bull 1983; 9(3): 371-5. t
[http://dx.doi.org/10.1177/0146167283093007]

[67] Healy E, Simpson N. Acne vulgaris. BMJ 1994; 308(6932): 831-3.
[http://dx.doi.org/10.1136/bmj.308.6932.831] [PMID: 8167492]

[68] Krowchuk DP, Stancin T, Keskinen R, Walker R, Bass J, Anglin TM. The psychosocial effects of acne on adolescents. Pediatr Dermatol 1991; 8(4): 332-8.
[http://dx.doi.org/10.1111/j.1525-1470.1991.tb00945.x] [PMID: 1838809]

[69] Rubinow DR, Peck GL, Squillace KM, Gantt GG. Reduced anxiety and depression in cystic acne patients after successful treatment with oral isotretinoin. J Am Acad Dermatol 1987; 17(1): 25-32.
[http://dx.doi.org/10.1016/S0190-9622(87)70166-2] [PMID: 2956296]

[70] Pochi PE, Shalita AR, Strauss JS, *et al.* Report of the consensus conference in acne classification. J Am Acad Dermatol 1991; 24(3): 495-500.
[http://dx.doi.org/10.1016/S0190-9622(08)80076-X] [PMID: 1829466]

[71] Lazarus RS. Coping theory and research: past, present, and future. Psychosom Med 1993; 55(3): 234-47.
[http://dx.doi.org/10.1097/00006842-199305000-00002] [PMID: 8346332]

[72] Shah RB. Psychological assessment intervention for people with skin disease. In: Bewley A, Taylor RE, Reichenberg JS, Magid M, Eds. Practical Psychodermatology. Chichester: John Wiley & Sons Ltd 2014; pp. 40-9.
[http://dx.doi.org/10.1002/9781118560648.ch5]

[73] Fried RD. Nonpharmacological treatments in psychodermatology. In: Koo JY, Lee CS, Eds. Psychocutaneous medicine. New York: Marcel Decker Inc 2003; pp. 411-26.

[74] Root S, Kent G, al-Abadie MS. The relationship between disease severity, disability and psychological distress in patients undergoing PUVA treatment for psoriasis. Dermatology (Basel) 1994; 189(3): 234-7.
[http://dx.doi.org/10.1159/000246844] [PMID: 7949473]

CHAPTER 4

Body Dysmorphic Disorder – Quick Guide to Diagnosis and Treatment

Diana Radu Djurfeldt*

Psykiatri Sydväst, M46, Karolinska University Hospital, Huddinge, Sweden

Abstract: Body dysmorphic disorder (BDD) is a psychiatric condition with onset in early teens. Incidence and chronicity are about the same as for schizophrenia or obsessive compulsive disorder affecting 1-2% of the population with a chronic progressive course in many cases. A higher prevalence has been noticed among girls. The insight is usually low. Next of kin are often affected by the patients distress and low functioning.

The etiology of BDD is partly explained genetically, partly associated to environmental factors such as abuse or neglect. Neurofunctional imaging and psychological tests reveal an imbalance between global versus local visual processing resulting in high focus on perceiving aberrant details.

Diagnosis of BDD has steadily improved over the last decades with new criteria recently published in the DSM 5. Comorbidity with depression, substance abuse or other anxiety disorders are common and the risk for suicide is high in this group.

Treatment consists of SSRI or clomipramine as first and second line medications. Glutamatergic agents, anticonvulsants and neuroleptic agents are currently studied in BDD. The psychological treatment of choice is cognitive behaviour therapy focusing on exposure and ritual prevention. The effects of treatment, medication, therapy or combined treatments are fairly good.

BDD is a common, severely debilitating disorder with early onset where treatment can improve the symptoms and quality of life. Recognising the diagnosis and providing relevant information give affected patients a fair chance to get qualified help.

Keywords: Body dysmorphic disorder, Buspirone, Cognitive behaviour therapy, Dysmorphophobia, Serotonine reuptake inhibitors.

* **Corresponding author Diana Radu Djurfeldt:** Psykiatri Sydväst, M46, Karolinska University Hospital, Huddinge, Sweden; Tel: 46-8-58585722; E-mail: Diana.Radu-Djurfeldt@sll.se.

Klas Nordlind & Anna Zalewska-Janowska (Eds.)

CASE STUDY

Lisa just turned 18. She is referred from child- and adolescent psychiatric unit to a specialist unit for OCD-spectrum disorders for further care.

Lisa has a long history of contacts with child psychiatry. Lisa has always been a good student but has missed a lot of schoolwork in high school because of home-sitting. She comes to her first appointment with her parents. Lisa is a quite normal looking girl wearing jeans, a collage jumper a bit too big, has sunglasses and a her hair covering parts of her face. She insists on sitting in a corner turned from the window.

Lisa seems reluctant to be in the doctor's office and most of her story is told by her parents. It appears that Lisa is a happy child who enjoyed playing with other kids. There were no complications during pregnancy or birth and Lisa has not had any injuries or serious diseases. Her problems started in early teens when she became increasingly preoccupied by her weight and body shape as some of her friends. By the age of 15, she developed anorexia and needed to be hospitalized for a period of some weeks. One year later, she was stable in keeping her BMI above 17 and did no longer fulfil the criteria for an eating disorder. Meanwhile she started to be increasingly concerned about her face. Lisa thinks her complexion is too pale and there are hideous red spots all over the face. She is bothered about her high cheekbones, the uneven hairline, the eyebrows and lips also. At the beginning, Lisa used to spend a lot of time scrutinizing her perceived flaws in the mirror; she took photos with her cell phone or looked in all reflecting areas such as car and shops windows to check her defects. Lately though, she rather avoids reflecting areas as the sight she sees is scary and makes her feel really depressed.

Lisa sought help for her spots from many dermatologists. She got some ointments but does not think it helped. She also spends time looking for a cure on internet and talks to other teens bothered about their complexion on blogs and forums. Lisa wants her parents to pay for dermabrasion and would also want to change the shape of the cheek bones and hair line by surgery but the expenses are high.

Lisa engages in time consuming rituals for treating her facial skin. Firstly, she used to go up one hour earlier to be in time for school but after some months the time needed for treatment, washing, camouflaging, picking the hair line and eyebrows perfectly increased steadily, so Lisa missed school anyway more and more often. She has not been to school more than a few days this last term as she is severely depressed by the thought of her appearance. She rarely leaves home and when doing so takes a lot of time to put on a thorough make up covering the blemishes, fixing the hair and putting on the right clothing to hide all the defects. The makeup needs to be done in a certain way and is the most time consuming part. It happens now more and more often that Lisa still feels disappointed in spite of the make up being done by all rules, and has to wash it all off and redo the process thoroughly. While out or at school, Lisa can see how others pity her for her horrible looks, which is utmost distressing. She is certain that some of her classmates even cry when they see her. Lisa cannot see how she would ever be able to feel better, not as long as the disgusting details in the face are not corrected surgically or by laser. She spends most of her time now on computer chatting or searching for information and cures. She loses hope and thinks a lot about death as an alternative to her severe suffering but assures you she does not want to harm herself and really wants help with her defects. However, the only interest she has in talking to a psychiatrist is to get a referral to plastic surgery to get help.

During her contact with child- and adolescent psychiatry, Lisa was reluctant to medication. She had regular contact with a therapist who tried to treat her for social phobia. However, Lisa did not think this would help and mostly sat off the sessions with quite low interest. She still does not think psychiatry can help but admits that treating her anorexia earlier actually did work and made her concern about weight go away.

BACKGROUND

Dysmorphophobia was described already in 1891 by Enrico Morselli as a phobic disorder focusing on fixation on the idea of one´s deformity. About a century later, in 1980, the term dysmorphophobia first made its entrance into the American Diagnostic and statistical manual DSM III among somatophorm disorders described as an ”atypical” one. In 1987, in the revised version DSM III-R [1], it changes name to Body Dysmorphic Disorder, the term currently in use [2,

3]. In the DSM IV [4], BDD still stays within the somatophorm subgroup. The high degree of similarities between BDD and obsessive compulsive disorder (OCD) with persistent thoughts related to perceived flaws in one's appearance together with ritualized repetitive behaviours made clinicians and researchers argue for including BDD in a new section of "Obsessive Compulsive and related disorders" in the DSM 5 [5] (Table **1**).

Table 1. Diagnostic criteria of BDD according to ICD 10 / DSM IV-TR / DSM 5.

Criterium	ICD 10 (F42.22)	DSM IV-TR (300.7)	DSM 5 (300.7)
A		Preoccupation with an imagined defect in appearance. If a slight physical anomaly is present, the person's concern is markedly excessive.	Preoccupation with one or more perceived defects or flaws in physical appearance that are not observable or appear slight to others.
B		The preoccupation causes clinically significant distress or impairment in social, occupational, or other important areas of functioning.	At some point during the course of the disorder, the individual has performed repetitive behaviours (*e.g.* mirror checking, excessive grooming, skin picking, reassurance seeking) or mental acts (*e.g.* comparing his or her appearance with that of others) in response to the appearance concerns.
C		The preoccupation is not better accounted for by another mental disorder (*e.g.*, dissatisfaction with body shape and size in Anorexia Nervosa).	The preoccupation causes clinical significant distress or impairment in social, occupational, or other important areas of functioning.
D			The appearance preoccupation is not better explained by concerns with body fat or weight in an individual whose symptoms meet criteria for an eating disorder.
Specify if:			With muscle dysmorphia With good or fair insight With poor insight With absent insight/delusional beliefs

At the same time, the ICD 10 (International statistical classification of diseases and related health problems) [6] still uses the term "dysmorphophobia", referring to it as a variant/example of hypochondriasis and not as a separate diagnosis.

However, in the revised version of the ICD 11, BDD will most probably be classified as a separate diagnosis in harmony with the classification of the DSM 5.

SYMPTOMATOLOGY

The most common feature a patient with BDD will be concerned about is a well-defined defect in the appearance. It can be spots on the face, asymmetry in facial features, size of the nose, angle of the eyes, quality or texture of the skin or hair, shades or transparency of the skin, size and shape of the breasts, height, shape of the head, the hairline, *etc.* The defect can readily be described by the patient with high precision and the dissatisfaction is rather persistent over time and causes often extensive distress, avoidance, and decrease in normal function. The patient engages in ritualized repeated behaviours similar to compulsions always aiming in BDD on diminishing or hiding the perceived defect such as checking, comparing, camouflaging, choosing to sit exposing the "good" side of the body/face, avoiding strong light/sun. Some patients check their appearance in all reflecting surfaces such as mirrors, car or shop windows, their cell phone, or even avoid reflecting areas. The degree of insight varies but tends to be low.

General unhappiness about one's appearance or generally feeling ugly/un-attractive should not be mistaken for BDD. In BDD, the patient is unhappy with very specific details in his/her appearance to such degree that the preoccupation interferes markedly with the possibility to live a normal life. The quality of the perception of this/these bodily defect/s in patients with BDD is similar in intensity to the erroneous body image characteristic for patients with eating disorders (anorexia) [7, 8].

AETIOLOGY AND PATHOGENESIS

BDD occurs both sporadic and in families. Environmental factors such as neglect and abuse increase the risk to develop BDD. Genetic factors explain around 44 % of the variance in different studies [9]. Incidence of BDD is also elevated in 1st relatives of individuals with OCD.

The disorder usually starts in early teens peaking at 13 years of age. Girls are more often affected than boys with a sexual difference in prevalence of 3:2

girls:boys. Untreated, BDD is a chronic disorder [10]. Comorbidity is common, many patients also have depressions (75%), alcohol-or drug abuse (up to 50%), social phobia (nearly 40%) and OCD (slightly above 30%). Persons with substance abuse see it as a form of self-medication as BDD symptoms in this group usually precedes substance abuse symptoms with at least one year [11]. Due to the severe decline in functioning and working capacity and low quality of life, the risk for suicidal ideation and behaviour is common in this group [12].

The incidence of BDD at dermatology clinics and at cosmetic dermatological consults is high ranging between 11- 25 % affecting mostly females aged 35-50 and men under the age of 35 [11]. Incidence among American and German students is about 4% of individual fulfilling the diagnostic criteria for BDD [3, 13 - 15].

Different theories attempt to explain the pathogenesis of BDD: Self-discrepancy has been suggested by Veale *et al.* [16] presenting in individuals with BDD as focusing on the contrast between the perceived actual self and the ideal image of self, thereby generating a high level of distress. Functional neuroanatomy studies reveal differences in perception in patients with BDD. The defects seen by these individuals are not "imagined" but seen as such. Functional imaging studies suggest increased focus on details parallel with a decreased capacity to process whole images [17, 18]. The abnormal brain activation pattern is of hypoactivity in brain association areas for holistic processing together with abnormal allocation of prefrontal systems for details. These aberrant patterns of activation are seen both in processing of appearance but also of other objects such as houses, findings consistent with an explanatory model of imbalance between global *versus* local visual processing, a pattern also seen in neuropsychological tests [18 - 20]. Tractography data suggests that the impairment in insight might be associated disorganization of neuronal connections between areas of visual and emotion/memory processing [21].

Perceptual abnormality involving several systems results in focusing on local details and missing global interpretation of visual input [17]. The visual system seems biased when interpreting emotions and patients with BDD more often interpret even neutral faces as angry or upset [22 - 24]. Speed of processing visual and emotional information seems decreased as compared to healthy controls, patients with BDD performing weaker in visuospatial tasks and in processing of emotional faces [22, 25 - 27]. Details improperly conceptualised may appear magnified or distorted.

DIAGNOSIS

Individuals with BDD will not primarily seek help from psychiatry but may turn up at the dermatologist, GP or at various "beauty clinics" asking for plastic surgery. These patients are quite often ashamed of their condition and afraid of not being taken seriously. If contacting psychiatry mostly for secondary comorbid disorders (mostly depression, social phobia, substance abuse, suicidal behaviour) [28], these patients will not self-report these BDD-symptoms. It is of great importance to find the underlying BDD in these cases by asking questions about e. g., anxiety in social situations and distress over details in the appearance and the impact of their symptoms on general function. Reassurance concerning the perceived flaws, on "looking good" will not help these patients and might even worsen their mistrust in healthcare.

As many patients also have eating disorders and avoid daylight, laboratory screening checking for anaemia, vitamin levels (cobalamine, folate and 25-OH-D-vitamin), thyroid tests among other routine analysis should be performed early after diagnosis.

Example of Screening Question

"Are you concerned about details in your appearance though others reassure you of looking fine?" and "Do you spend much time trying to hide this perceived flaw in your appearance or spend much time checking it or thinking of it?" DSM 5 offers a screening scales to use when suspecting BDD, the BDD-D (BDD Dimensional Scale) [29].

If the screening questions are positive, further questions should be asked following the diagnostic criteria in the DSM 5. Also, questions about depressive symptoms and suicidality should be addressed due to high co-morbidity.

The gold standard in following outcome of BDD treatment is the Yale Brown

Obsessive Compulsive Scale modified for BDD (BDD-YBOCS). The BDD-YBOCS is a clinician rated scale to assess the severity of BDD symptoms consisting of 12 items ranging from 0 to 48 [30]. The scale is built in a parallel way addressing thoughts (items 1-5), behaviours (items 6-10) related to BDD as well as insight (item 11) and avoidance (item 12), all items scoring 0-4.

TREATMENT

Serotonergic agents have been proven effective as medication in BDD. Selective serotonin reuptake inhibitors (SSRI) are the first line recommended treatment alternative [31]. The dosage should be increased to the highest tolerable level aiming for the highest dose recommended for the respective drug. Clomipramine, a tricyclic antidepressant agent with serotonergic profile should be tried in case other treatments failed. The serotonin partial agonist, buspirone, in doses of 50-60 mg/day, also has some evidence in the treatment repertoire of BDD [32]. Atypical neuroleptics as adjuvants to SRI's have so far not proven helpful, however the studies to date are small [33]. Trials with other agents affecting glutamate and dopamine systems are on-going with case reports of beneficial effect of agents such as anticonvulsants [34]. There is no evidence in using sedatives /hypnotics such as benzodiazepines in the treatment of BDD. The negative effect on cognitive functions diminishing the possibility in attending CBT together with the risk for substance abuse should be carefully addressed even if intermittent doses are enquired for.

CBT is the psychological treatment alternative of choice where combination with pharmacotherapy should be encouraged, especially as untreated depressions might interfere with the possibility for patients to engage in CBT. The most important "ingredient" in CBT for BDD is exposure, prolonged and repeated, to feared situations together with ritual prevention, *i.e.* restraining from camouflage, grooming, seeking reassurance, *etc.* when doing the exposure training.

Exposure to mirror checking is another common ingredient in CBT-techniques for BDD, however many patients do not show habituation to mirroring, possibly explained by the decreased set-shifting capacity and impaired visual and emotional processing resulting in frontostriatal systems unable to inhibit subcortical areas. The goals of CBT are restoring the earlier decrease in function. The patients own striving to acquire future goals stays in discrepancy to the extended avoidance behaviour he/she has been practising to reduce discomfort and is a key motivator for changes in behaviour.

As many patients have poor or no insight, treatment motivation may be low and treatment failure is a common problem. The clinician should keep motivating the patient and be available for new trials as periods of ambivalence might precede later good treatment outcome. Earlier CBT should be carefully assessed in chronic cases where rational for exposure, ritual prevention, repeated exposure as home works between sessions and intensity of treatment with sessions occurring weekly should be asked for. Therapist led exposure might be important for some patients with severe symptoms who are not able to commit to the treatment on their own. More intensive treatment could be administered as an in-patient program if so needed.

The BDD-YBOCS is a good way to follow treatment response or disorder progress/relapse together with depression rating scales and assessment of function level at work as well as in social and family life.

A majority of BDD-patients benefit from SSRI and CBT. Giving hope, relevant information and the possibility to seek qualified help even after initial ambivalence is crucial in the care of individuals with BDD.

CONFLICT OF INTEREST

The author confirms that they have no conflict of interest to declare for this publication.

ACKNOWLEDGEMENTS

The fruitful discussions with Jesper Enade, psychotherapist and researcher at Karolinska Insitutet, are gratefully acknowledged.

REFERENCES

[1] American Psychiatric Association. Diagnostic and statistical manual of mental disorders Washington, DC 1980.

[2] Altamura C, Paluello MM, Mundo E, Medda S, Mannu P. Clinical and subclinical body dysmorphic disorder. Eur Arch Psychiatry Clin Neurosci 2001; 251(3): 105-8. [http://dx.doi.org/10.1007/s004060170042] [PMID: 11697569]

[3] Phillips KA. Body dysmorphic disorder: diagnostic controversies and treatment challenges. Bull Menninger Clin 2000; 64(1): 18-35. [PMID: 10695157]

[4] American Psychiatric Association. Diagnostic and statistical manual of mental disorders Washington, DC 1994.

[5] American Psychiatric Association. DSM-5 Task Force, Diagnostic and statistical manual of mental disorders: Washington, DC 2013; p. xliv: 947.

[6] The ICD-10 classification of mental and behavioural disorders: clinical descriptions and diagnostic guidelines. Geneva : World Health Organization 1992; p. xii, 362.

[7] Feusner JD, Townsend J, Bystritsky A, Bookheimer S. Visual information processing of faces in body dysmorphic disorder. Arch Gen Psychiatry 2007; 64(12): 1417-25. [http://dx.doi.org/10.1001/archpsyc.64.12.1417] [PMID: 18056550]

[8] Madsen SK, Bohon C, Feusner JD. Visual processing in anorexia nervosa and body dysmorphic disorder: similarities, differences, and future research directions. J Psychiatr Res 2013; 47(10): 1483-91. [http://dx.doi.org/10.1016/j.jpsychires.2013.06.003] [PMID: 23810196]

[9] Monzani B, Rijsdijk F, Anson M, *et al.* A twin study of body dysmorphic concerns. Psychol Med 2012; 42(9): 1949-55. [http://dx.doi.org/10.1017/S0033291711002741] [PMID: 22126745]

[10] Phillips KA, Menard W, Quinn E, Didie ER, Stout RL. A 4-year prospective observational follow-up study of course and predictors of course in body dysmorphic disorder. Psychol Med 2013; 43(5): 1109-17. [http://dx.doi.org/10.1017/S0033291712001730] [PMID: 23171833]

[11] Phillips KA, Menard W, Fay C, Weisberg R. Demographic characteristics, phenomenology, comorbidity, and family history in 200 individuals with body dysmorphic disorder. Psychosomatics 2005; 46(4): 317-25. [http://dx.doi.org/10.1176/appi.psy.46.4.317] [PMID: 16000674]

[12] Phillips KA, Menard W. Suicidality in body dysmorphic disorder: a prospective study. Am J Psychiatry 2006; 163(7): 1280-2. [http://dx.doi.org/10.1176/ajp.2006.163.7.1280] [PMID: 16816236]

[13] Oosthuizen P, Lambert T, Castle DJ. Dysmorphic concern: prevalence and associations with clinical variables. Aust N Z J Psychiatry 1998; 32(1): 129-32. [http://dx.doi.org/10.3109/00048679809062719] [PMID: 9565194]

[14] Bohne A, Wilhelm S, Keuthen NJ, Florin I, Baer L, Jenike MA. Prevalence of body dysmorphic disorder in a German college student sample. Psychiatry Res 2002; 109(1): 101-4. [http://dx.doi.org/10.1016/S0165-1781(01)00363-8] [PMID: 11850057]

[15] Otto MW, Wilhelm S, Cohen LS, Harlow BL. Prevalence of body dysmorphic disorder in a community sample of women. Am J Psychiatry 2001; 158(12): 2061-3. [http://dx.doi.org/10.1176/appi.ajp.158.12.2061] [PMID: 11729026]

[16] Veale D, Kinderman P, Riley S, Lambrou C. Self-discrepancy in body dysmorphic disorder. Br J Clin Psychol 2003; 42(Pt 2): 157-69. [http://dx.doi.org/10.1348/014466503321903571] [PMID: 12828805]

[17] Monzani B, Krebs G, Anson M, Veale D, Mataix-Cols D. Holistic *versus* detailed visual processing in body dysmorphic disorder: testing the inversion, composite and global precedence effects. Psychiatry Res 2013; 210(3): 994-9. [http://dx.doi.org/10.1016/j.psychres.2013.08.009] [PMID: 23993467]

[18] Feusner JD, Hembacher E, Moller H, Moody TD. Abnormalities of object visual processing in body dysmorphic disorder. Psychol Med 2011; 41(11): 2385-97. [http://dx.doi.org/10.1017/S0033291711000572] [PMID: 21557897]

[19] Arienzo D, Leow A, Brown JA, *et al.* Abnormal brain network organization in body dysmorphic disorder. Neuropsychopharmacology 2013; 38(6): 1130-9. [http://dx.doi.org/10.1038/npp.2013.18] [PMID: 23322186]

[20] Kerwin L, Hovav S, Hellemann G, Feusner JD. Impairment in local and global processing and set-shifting in body dysmorphic disorder. J Psychiatr Res 2014; 57: 41-50. [http://dx.doi.org/10.1016/j.jpsychires.2014.06.003] [PMID: 24972487]

[21] Feusner JD, Arienzo D, Li W, *et al.* White matter microstructure in body dysmorphic disorder and its clinical correlates. Psychiatry Res 2013; 211(2): 132-40. [http://dx.doi.org/10.1016/j.pscychresns.2012.11.001] [PMID: 23375265]

[22] Feusner JD, Bystritsky A, Hellemann G, Bookheimer S. Impaired identity recognition of faces with emotional expressions in body dysmorphic disorder. Psychiatry Res 2010; 179(3): 318-23. [http://dx.doi.org/10.1016/j.psychres.2009.01.016] [PMID: 20493560]

[23] Buhlmann U, McNally RJ, Etcoff NL, Tuschen-Caffier B, Wilhelm S. Emotion recognition deficits in body dysmorphic disorder. J Psychiatr Res 2004; 38(2): 201-6. [http://dx.doi.org/10.1016/S0022-3956(03)00107-9] [PMID: 14757335]

[24] Buhlmann U, Etcoff NL, Wilhelm S. Emotion recognition bias for contempt and anger in body dysmorphic disorder. J Psychiatr Res 2006; 40(2): 105-11. [http://dx.doi.org/10.1016/j.jpsychires.2005.03.006] [PMID: 15904932]

[25] Jefferies K, Laws KR, Fineberg N. Superior face recognition in body dysmorphic disorder. J Psychopharmacol 2011; 25(8): A48.

[26] Deckersbach T, Savage CR, Phillips KA, *et al.* Characteristics of memory dysfunction in body dysmorphic disorder. J Int Neuropsychol Soc 2000; 6(6): 673-81. [http://dx.doi.org/10.1017/S1355617700666055] [PMID: 11011514]

[27] Yaryura-Tobias JA, Neziroglu F, Chang R, Lee S, Pinto A, Donohue L. Computerized perceptual analysis of patients with body dysmorphic disorder: a pilot study. CNS Spectr 2002; 7(6): 444-6. [PMID: 15107766]

[28] Phillips KA, Siniscalchi JM, McElroy SL. Depression, anxiety, anger, and somatic symptoms in patients with body dysmorphic disorder. Psychiatr Q 2004; 75(4): 309-20. [http://dx.doi.org/10.1023/B:PSAQ.0000043507.03596.0d] [PMID: 15563049]

[29] LeBeau RM, Simpson H, Mataix-Cols D, Phillips KA, Stein D, Craske M. Preliminary assessment of obsessive ?"compulsive spectrum disorder scales for DSM-5. J Obsessive-Compulsive Relat Disord 2013; 2: 114-8. [http://dx.doi.org/10.1016/j.jocrd.2013.01.005]

[30] Phillips KA, Hollander E, Rasmussen SA, Aronowitz BR, DeCaria C, Goodman WK. A severity rating scale for body dysmorphic disorder: development, reliability, and validity of a modified version of the Yale-Brown Obsessive Compulsive Scale. Psychopharmacol Bull 1997; 33(1): 17-22. [PMID: 9133747]

[31] Phillips KA, Hollander E. Treating body dysmorphic disorder with medication: evidence, misconceptions, and a suggested approach. Body Image 2008; 5(1): 13-27. [http://dx.doi.org/10.1016/j.bodyim.2007.12.003] [PMID: 18325859]

[32] Phillips KA. An open study of buspirone augmentation of serotonin-reuptake inhibitors in body dysmorphic disorder. Psychopharmacol Bull 1996; 32(1): 175-80. [PMID: 8927669]

[33] Rashid H, Khan AA, Fineberg NA. Adjunctive antipsychotic in the treatment of body dysmorphic disorder - A retrospective naturalistic case note study. Int J Psychiatry Clin Pract 2015; 19(2): 84-9. [PMID: 25363200]

[34] Wang HR, Woo YS, Bahk WM. Potential role of anticonvulsants in the treatment of obsessive-compulsive and related disorders. Psychiatry Clin Neurosci 2014; 68(10): 723-32. [http://dx.doi.org/10.1111/pcn.12186] [PMID: 24735021]

CHAPTER 5

Skin Picking Disorders and Dermatitis Artefacta

Anthony Bewley[1,2,*] and **Padma Mohandas**[1]

[1] *Departments of Dermatology, Whipps Cross University Hospital, London, UK*

[2] *The Royal London Hospital, London, UK*

Abstract: Dermatologists and patients have long known that skin diseases affect the physical and emotional well-being of a person's existence. Conversely, the psychological state of a person can also affect his/her skin. In this chapter, we set out the nature and basis of some of the dermatological conditions linked to obsessive compulsive disorders [SPD and Acne excoriee] and also take a look at Dermatitis Artefacta, a poorly understood factitious disorder. We present the process of evaluation and care of this vulnerable group of patients, whilst also highlighting the importance of a holistic approach in a multidisciplinary setting.

The skin is well placed to be the focus of tension reducing and emotion regulating behaviours [1]. High levels of anxiety, in dissociative and obsessive compulsive states is perhaps one of the most significant influences in conditions such as Skin picking disorders [SPD] and Dermatitis Artefacta [DA]. Anxiety can also exacerbate primary skin disorders such as Acne with the development of Acne excoriee.

We know that psychological, psychiatric and psychosocial stress affect over 30% of dermatological patients. Assessment of these co-morbidities is therefore imperative in the overall clinical evaluation of the patient. Therefore an integrated multidisciplinary team approach to manage this group of patients leads to better outcomes.

Keywords: Acne excoriee, Artefactual, Compulsive, Dermatitis artefacta, Dermatology, Dissociation, DSM-5, Excoriation, Multidisciplinary team, Neurotic, Obsessive, Picking, Psychiatric, Psychodermatology, Psychosomatic, Skin.

* **Corresponding author Anthony Bewley:** Departments of Dermatology, Whipps Cross University Hospital, and The Royal London Hospital, London, UK; Tel: (+44)208 539 5522 ext 5248; Fax:(+44)208 535 6897; E-mail:anthony.bewley@bartshealth.nhs.uk.

Klas Nordlind & Anna Zalewska-Janowska (Eds.)

SKIN PICKING DISORDER

Synonyms

Psychogenic/Neurotic excoriation, Compulsive or Pathological skin picking, Dermatotillomania.

Key Features

- Most prevalent in middle aged women (30-50 years).
- Intense desire to pick/rub or scratch real or imagined lesions.
- Sites affected are usually easily accessible such as the face, upper back, extensors of arms and legs, genitalia and buttocks.
- Anxiety and depression are strongly associated co-morbidities.

Introduction

As many as one fifth of the general population admit to skin picking that result in tissue disruption. Clinically significant SPD however ranges from 5-8% and is characterised by repetitive and compulsive picking of the skin resulting in tissue damage. Patients feel the urge to disturb the skin and find relief in the activity. Attempts to suppress the urge can cause an increase in psychological tension. The picking may begin inadvertently or manifest in a ritualistic fashion. Certain situations may trigger the picking such as looking into a mirror, being alone or stressed. The picking behaviour may be followed by feelings of gratification, relief or pleasure [2].

Some individuals may engage in more automatic picking, which occurs without full awareness of the patient and devoid of any preceding tension. In such circumstances, there tends to be higher levels of emotional dysregulation. This dissociative component is important to recognise, as these patients need stabilisation and a risk assessment for suicide.

Epidemiology

The true extent of this disorder is unknown as few studies have been conducted as to the overall incidence of SPD, however, there is an 8% prevalence in the psycho dermatology setting. Interpretation of these prevalence rates is complicated by the fact that SPD may be a manifestation of other disorders such as Obsessive Compulsive Disorder (OCD) (to remove contaminants), genetic disorders like Prader Willi syndrome and Body Dysmorphic Disorder (BDD). Although the condition can present at any age, the peak ages of presentation seem to be between 30 to 50 years. There is a distinct female preponderance.

Clinical Features

Lesions may arise from pre-existing skin problems like acne or urticated papules or they may be created *de–novo.* Research conducted by Wilhelm *et al.* [3] showed that the most common sites of involvement were the face (Fig. **1**) and back, the "butterfly sign" is a distinctive feature whereby the inability of the patient to reach the central areas of the back results in peripheral skin trauma resembling that of butterfly wings [4]. Many patients use their fingernails to pick or squeeze lesions. A significant number also use implements such as tweezers and needles. Lesions may range in size from a few millimetres to several centimetres. In extreme cases of SPD, the individual may gouge as deep as the muscle and arteries. Morphologies vary from superficial erosions to deep ulceration. Post inflammatory hypo or hyper pigmentation is common. On the scalp, there may be broken hairs or areas of alopecia. Women may sometimes report worsening of symptoms pre-menstrually.

Psychiatrically, these patients are a heterogeneous group most commonly expressing obsessive compulsive traits [5]. In some, picking may be an expression of a generalised anxiety disorder or depression. When stressed or tensed there may be anxious and restless picking at any interruption on the surface of the skin, with the activity frequently occurring at night or when the patient is unoccupied [6]. Psychosocial stressors must therefore be enquired upon when taking the history.

From a psycho dynamic perspective, there are often histories of difficult childhoods with emotional rejection and harsh parenting. Individuals may lack self-confidence and be overly sensitive to criticism. A percentage also have anger management issues which is displaced into self-destructive picking.

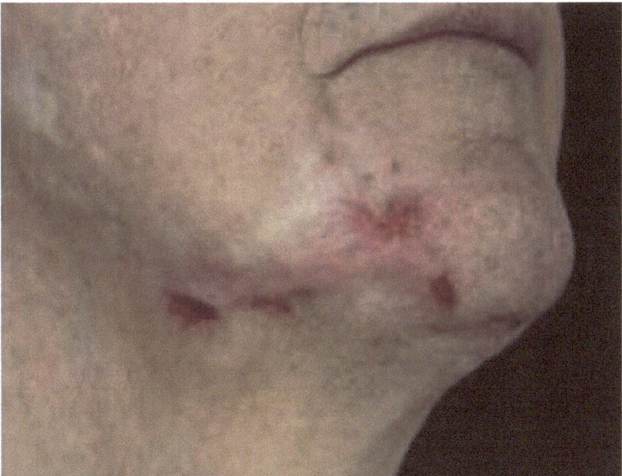

Fig. (1). Skin picking disorder affecting the face. Note excoriations, ulceration and scarring at the same site.

Differential Diagnosis

The differentials should include both medical and psychiatric conditions. Medical causes for itching that can induce excoriation include urticaria, uraemia, cholestatic hepatitis, scabies, lichen planus (look for oral lesions), xerosis, cutaneous dysesthesia, malignancies and if predominantly photo distributed it is important to exclude photosensitive disorders such as actinic prurigo and porphyria cutanea tarda. Psychiatric conditions that can lead to excoriating behaviour include anxiety, depression, OCD, body dysmorphic disorder, delusional infestation, borderline personality disorder, dermatitis artefacta and somatoform disorders, such as hypochondriasis. Recreational drug use like cocaine and cannabis should also be enquired upon as well as alcohol consumption.

Investigations

Physical causes of pruritus and skin disease should be looked for and excluded in the first instance. See Box **1**.

Box 1. Suggested investigations for Skin picking disorder.

- **Blood tests** [Full Blood Count /Thyroid Function Test/Liver Function Test /Renal Function Test /Iron/Ferritin/Glucose], HIV serology and protein electrophoresis as clinically indicated.
- **Skin swabs** for microscopy and culture.
- **Skin biopsies with immunofluorescence** if needed.
- **Other tests** such as Chest X –ray/CT scans depending on the situation for suspected malignancies.

Management

Where possible, patients presenting with SPD /Acne excoriee should be managed in a dedicated psycho dermatology clinic, with the input of not only a dermatologist and psychiatrist but also with access to a psychologist and dermatology nurse specialist. Assessment of psychosocial morbidities such as psychological trauma and stressful life events are important, as these factors have shown to have a direct impact on skin barrier function and immune response [7]. There are numerous disease specific SPS-Skin Picking Scale, Y-BOCS-Yale Brown Obsessive Compulsive Scale and general quality of life scales such as the DLQI (Dermatology Life Quality Index) and HAD (Hospital Anxiety and Depression) that assess stress and the impact on the skin. They are useful as an objective measure of evaluating health related quality of life, in adults suffering from skin problems. When managing these patients it is good practice to combine both the dermatological and psychiatric evaluation together. Our experience of evaluation in a joint psycho-dermatology clinic is that psychiatric assessment can be conducted progressively over time. The patient's issues are viewed holistically from the outset, with rapport building between the patient and dermatologist and psychiatrist as sessions unfold.

1. Communication

As with all psycho dermatological conditions patients should be dealt with in a non – confrontational manner. Fostering a positive relationship by empathising with their condition is important. It may also be helpful to explain that although the actual reason for their symptoms is not clearly understood, there are strategies that can be employed which can change the way the skin and brain process the signals it receives.

2. Treatment of Skin Picking Disorder

a. Topical

Treatment is based on symptom severity. For example, if pruritus is an issue, preparations of Menthol containing emollients may be useful *e.g.* in Menthol in Aqueous Cream or 5% Doxepin cream. Cool compresses can be helpful to remove crusting and to soothe the skin. Emollients patient preference to be considered with or without antiseptics can also be suggested to improve hydration, and thereby reducing sensation of itch. A point to note is that adopting a positive approach in dealing with skin issues helps enormously as patients invariably become upset if the cutaneous component of their condition is overlooked.

Topical/Intralesional steroids/tape to address the inflammatory component of existing lesions can be used as adjunct for chronic or non healing lesions. Combinations of antibiotics and glucocorticoids [Fucibet] can also be applied in a tapering dose over days or weeks.

b. Systemic Therapy

[i]. Physical

Phototherapy [TL01] whole body or localised, can be used with good results especially in cases where widespread itching is a feature. The mechanism of action is through the immunomodulatory and anti-inflammatory effects of phototherapy which leads to itch reduction and improvement of the underlying dermatitis.

[ii]. Pharmacotherapeutics

Antibiotics from the tetracycline group Lymecycline or Doxycycline have been tried with benefit where there may be a perceived infectious component to symptoms. Tetracyclines may be preferred for their anti-inflammatory as well as antibiotic effects. Treatment courses tend to last for weeks or months depending on the response. Conventional sedative antihistamines such as Hydroxyzine or Chlorpheneramine maleate [Piriton] can help with itching. The antipruritic effects of Doxepin may be particularly beneficial for patients with associated depression and anxiety. It can be given in doses of between 10-20 mg in the elderly, and up to 75-100 mg in younger patients.

3. Psychological and Psychiatric Interventions

a. Non Pharmacological Therapy

Counselling can be beneficial in those patients who have psychosocial stressors that have precipitated, or are perpetuating their skin problem *e.g.* bullying at school, marriage breakdown, bereavement. Cognitive behavioural therapy [CBT] can be very effective for patients with signs and symptoms of OCD, and who are willing to engage with their psychologist. It involves tailored treatment according to the individual needs of the patient.

b. Pharmacological Therapy

Obsessive compulsive symptoms as seen in skin picking disorders are associated with Serotonin mediated neural pathways. Antidepressants that selectively block serotonin uptake [SSRI's] can be of benefit in patients with this problem. Commonly used SSRI's include Citalopram, Sertraline and Fluoxetine. Mirtazipine, a noradrenergic and specific serotonergic antidepressant [NaSSA] is used primarily in the treatment of depression and has anxiolytic and sedative effects. Mirtazipine has a place on the therapeutic ladder where either the patient cannot tolerate SSRI's or where insomnia is a key feature.

Prognosis

This depends on:

1. The predisposing factors, for example a pre morbid anxious personality, other personality disorder or childhood traumas, physical or emotional abuse.
2. Precipitants such as stressful life events *e.g.* job loss, marital stress or bereavement.
3. Perpetuating factors *e.g.* unemployment, poverty and, social isolation.

The average duration of illness is reported to be around 5-8 years [8] with relapses and remissions that parallel stressful situations.

ACNE EXCORIÉE

Synonyms

Acne excoriee des jeunes filles

Key Features

- Thought to be a subset of SPD
- Seen in younger women
- Patients pick at real or imagined acne form lesions

Introduction

Acne excoriee is a self inflicted skin condition which is thought of as a subset of SPD where the picking or scratching is directed at real or imagined acne lesions. The condition differs from other artefactual dermatoses in that the patient usually admits the self inflicted nature of the condition. Social embarrassment prevents up to half of patients from seeking help. When managing this group of patients the mechanism of picking is usually not stressed upon, as it is the underlying psychosocial issue that is of importance. Given the high co-morbidity of skin picking with other psychiatric disorders, clinicians should enquire about the cutaneous and psychiatric symptoms when either is found to be present. Acne excoriee is most often seen in young women hence the description "des jeunes filles".

Epidemiology

Acne excoriee is not an uncommon diagnosis made in the psycho dermatology setting, comprising around 5% of patients seen. Many are women in their thirties who may have significant social co-morbidities.

Clinical Features

Individuals with acne excoriee usually [though not always] have some form of acne existing on the face, chest or back. Lesions can range from superficial excoriations (Fig. **2**) to deep gouges. Scarring, post inflammatory hyper and hypo pigmentation are common. As in other SPD's women may report pre-menstrual flare of their lesions and picking habits. Many patients have underlying anxiety and or depression as co-morbidities. Other psychiatric diagnoses to consider are Post Traumatic Stress Disorder [PTSD], Obsessive Compulsive Disorder [OCD] and Body Dysmorphic Disorder [BDD].

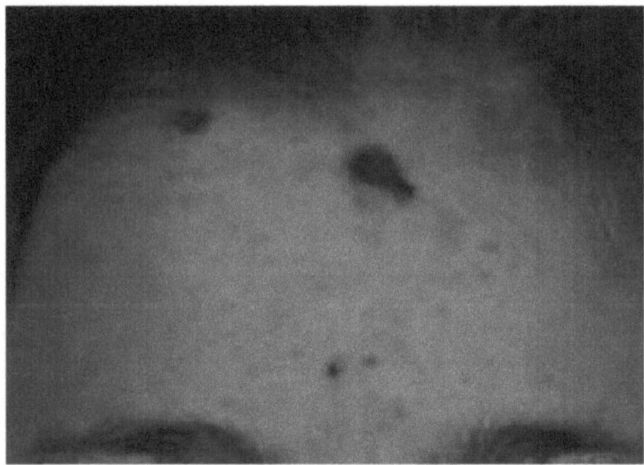

Fig. (2). Patient with mild acne and excoriated lesions on forehead.

Management

1. Treatment of Skin Disease

(a). Topical Treatments

The most common treatment modalities for the skin include topical antibiotics [Duac/Zineryt], topical retinoids in singular or combination therapy [9]. Antiseptic washes may also be used as an adjunct.

(b). Systemic Therapy

For mild to moderate papulopustular acne, oral antibiotics can be useful. Anti-androgen treatment, Spironolactone and anti-androgen contraceptives such as Dianette are considered for pre-menstrual flares in women. Low doses of isotretinoin less than 0.5mg/kg body weight over a period of 12-18 months may be beneficial in *selected* cases with concomitant psychological/psychiatric input.

2. Psychological and Psychiatric Interventions

(a). Non Pharmacological Therapy

Addressing the psychosocial aspect of this condition is paramount given that anxiety and depression is the largest co-morbidities associated with acne excoriee. Counselling and CBT as mentioned previously have pivotal roles in helping the patient recover from their illness.

(b). Pharmacotherapy

SSRI's remain the cornerstone of management for patients with associated anxiety and depression. A simple screening tool like the HAD can help objectively assess which of the two exist, or predominate. It takes between 2-5 minutes to complete.

Scoring: Possible scores range from 0 to 21 for each subscale. An analysis of scores on the two subscales divides each mood state into four ranges: 'mild cases' [scores 8-res 8-10], 'moderate cases' [scores 11-res 11-15], and 'severe cases' [scores 16 or higher].

Citalopram may be preferred for the treatment of anxiety /depression in adults. Dosing starts at 10 mg od and increments [up to 40 mg od] depend on response to treatment. Fluoxetine is particularly useful in depressive disorders and OCD dosing starts at 20 mg up to a maximum of 60 mg once daily. Sertraline can be used for the same in both adults and children. In the paediatric population we would recommend the input of a child psychiatrist to initiate and monitor response. Other antidepressant like Amitriptyline and Mirtazipine also have a place in the management of this disorder, each agent should be prescribed on a case by case basis.

Prognosis

There are no accurate statistics regarding the outcomes of SPD/Acne excoriee. Experience however suggests that patients have good outcomes if managed in a multi-disciplinary team setting.

DERMATITIS ARTEFACTA

Synonyms

Artefactual skin disease, factitious dermatitis

Key Features

- Deliberately inflicted skin lesions
- Seen on accessible parts of the body
- May be produced consciously or in a dissociative state
- More commonly seen in women

Introduction

Dermatitis artefacta [DA] is a factitious disorder whereby skin lesions are produced deliberately by the patient. The patient may not be fully aware of this behaviour, and the true extent of this disorder is unknown. There is usually a relevant psychological or psychosocial element to their history. The patient may be aware that they are driven to create the lesions, or in some instances the activity may occur in a dissociative state outside the patients' awareness [10]. DA patients do not readily admit to producing their lesions and as a rule conceal the activity. There is a strong psychological component to the multifactorial aetiology of DA. Management of these patients can be especially challenging as many fail to engage effectively with their dermatologist [11].There are some subtle differences between DA and other factitious skin disorders. In DA the primary aim is to obtain attention and sympathy, in contrast to malingering, where the patient consciously fabricates illness for external [material] gains. Patients who exhibit deliberate self harm, intentionally injure themselves using their behaviour as a coping mechanism to relieve emotional distress whereas in DA the production of lesions often exist in a dissociative state.

Epidemiology

DA is a rare condition with an incidence of around 1/3000 patients seen in a general dermatology clinic. However, in a specialist psycho dermatology setting, around 1 in 20 are diagnosed with this condition. The vast majority of patients are female with age of onset ranging from 13-70 years.

Clinical Features

DA can mimic a wide range of dermatoses and is one facet of the whole picture of factitious skin disease. The condition, quite often will have been presented to various other clinicians. Patients are known to present with a collection of normal investigations and a bag full of ineffective medication. Lesions may be solitary or multiple, unilateral or symmetrical.

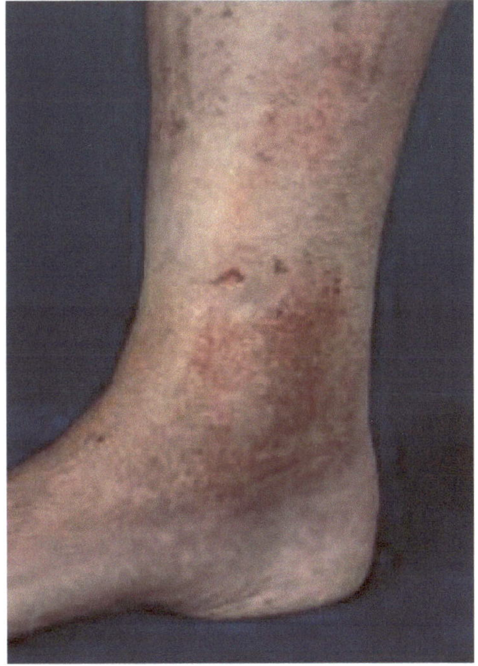

Fig. (3). Dermatitis artefacta – patient with erosions and nail lesions on legs.

Superficial erosion, excoriations (Figs. **3** and **4**) and post inflammatory pigmentation are the most common type of lesions observed. Blistering, purpura, ulceration and oedema are also observed. The morphology may appear quite bizarre in shape and distribution, appear on normal skin, and be angulated, geometric or streaky if corrosive liquids have been used, giving rise to the characteristic "drip sign". Chronic indolent lesions may prove more of a diagnostic challenge. The skin may have the appearance of a panniculitis and can be as a result of injection of substances into the skin. Lesions are often observed in areas which correspond to the side of hand dominance. The well-documented "hollow history" [12] , or inability of the patient to give details of the evolution of the lesions, is a characteristic feature of DA. All lesions appear to be at the same stage of development with little or no evidence of a "prodromal" phase [13]. The patients themselves may be remarkably unmoved by their condition, in contrast to accompanying family members who are often anxious and upset at what they perceive as medical incompetence.

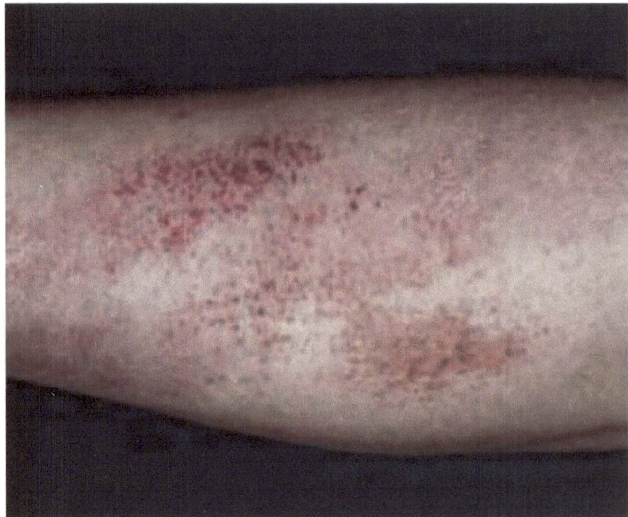

Fig. (4). Showing same patient with superficial excoriations on legs.

Psychosocial stressors must be elicited. In children bullying, exam stress, parental divorce or separation are the common precipitating factors. DA in this group is usually transient and milder, probably reflecting a maladaptive response to life events [14]. Patients whose life experiences were characterised by emotional deprivation are more likely to have an unstable body image, their relationships can be dependant and manipulative [15]. Chronic DA, may also be a manifestation of a disorder of body image associated with eating disorders [16]. Munchhausen's syndrome by proxy deserves a mention in that, it is the parent who is the patient, and the child who presenting with the problem may be too apprehensive to say otherwise.

Differential Diagnosis

In terms of differentials other than primary dermatological conditions, DA must be diagnosed from other psychiatric disorders presenting with skin features Delusional infestation, Neurotic excoriations, and malingering. The latter is characterised by self-inflicted lesions caused for a conscious gain. The most common primary skin disorders to consider are vasculitis, pyoderma gangrenosum, granulomatous skin disease and arthropod bites.

Investigations

These are mainly conducted to rule out primary dermatological conditions. Skin cultures can identify any secondary infection. A biopsy can help to ascertain the depth of the lesion and tissue reactions and perhaps also given the clinician a clue as to the causative agent which can in turn support the diagnosis of DA.

Management

Patients with DA present with diverse range of skin lesions, often with a psychosocial trigger. It is therefore essential for the clinician to explore *why* the patient is presenting with DA rather than *how* they are creating their skin lesions. A history of physical or sexual abuse may be elicited if there is involvement of the breast or genital area. We advocate a non-confrontational approach whilst managing patients with DA. Rather than focussing on the "surface" symptoms time is better spent understanding the "core issue" or reasons for the behaviour. To improve outcomes the emphasis should be to develop a strong patient –physician-family relationship. Therefore, there are two important objectives to achieve whilst managing patients with DA. Firstly, attempts should be made to respect appointment schedules and limit investigations to a minimum. Secondly it must be recognised that patients are in a way calling for help by self inflicting the lesions. Thus, it is imperative that a safe and accepting environment is created during the consultation [17]. One way of addressing their problems is to avoid any reference to the physical mechanism causing the lesions, instead focusing on the "stress" as the probable underlying factor, which may be easier for the patient to accept. Conversely it may be useful to address the fact that the illness itself is causing the stress and to use this rationale for the introduction of psychotherapy or a psychiatric consultation.

Dermatological Therapy

Conventional skin therapy such as topical antibacterial washes Dermol 500 or Octenisan and emollients may be prescribed depending on the presenting lesions. It is useful to prescribe these as it gives the patient some satisfaction that "something is being done" and may also replace the destructive behaviours causing the lesions in the first place. Occlusion has been used historically as a therapeutic and diagnostic aide [18]. However, patients may displace activities to other areas of skin if they do not feel secure or cared for. Table **1** illustrates the process of management in the U.K.

Table 1. Algorithm for managing patients presenting with DA.

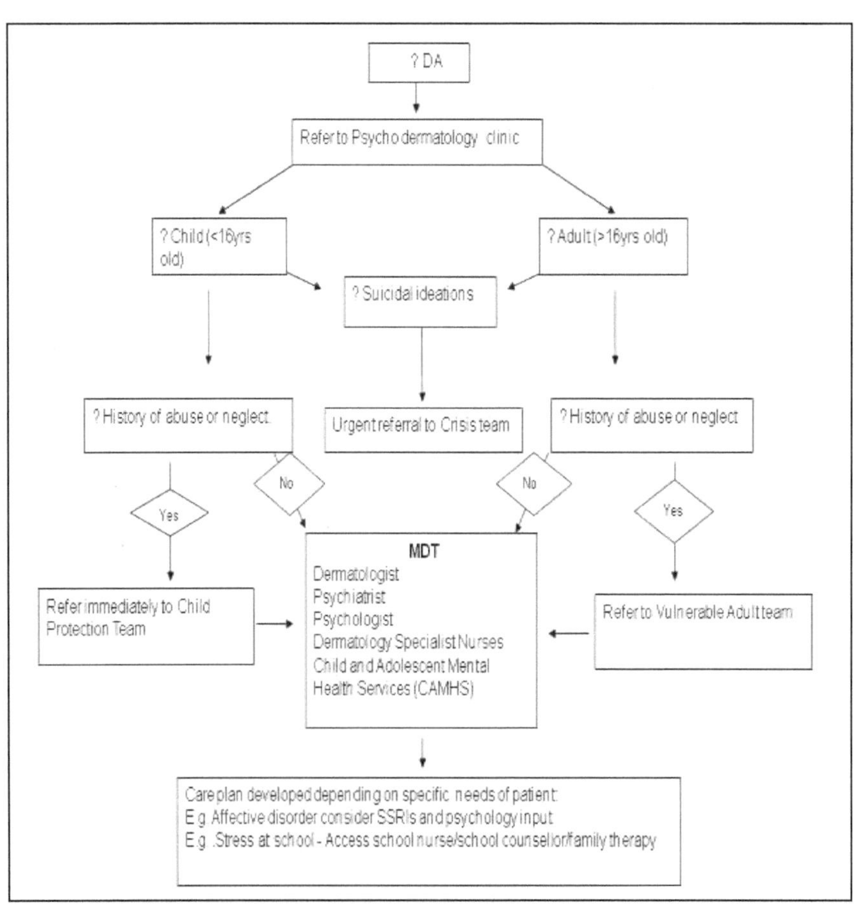

Psychiatric/Psychosocial Interventions

Treatment of the emotional components of DA includes both psycho-pharmacological and psychological approaches. In isolation, Psychotherapy and Cognitive behaviour therapy have varying degrees of success. Patients presenting to the dermatologist are often unwilling to accept the psychiatric nature of the disorder and lack the awareness of their circumstances that trigger the drive to produce the lesions. Hence the need for a combined approach.

Serotonin pathways are implicated in anxiety, depression and obsessive-compulsive disorders [19], it is also understood that serotonin pathways are involved in self injurious behaviour. Therefore, Selective Serotonin Uptake Inhibitors (SSRIs) can be used where there is an obsessive compulsive element to the self injury in DA, and also to treat any depressive or anxiety disorders. Low dose antipsychotics [20] like Risperidone, [starting at 0.5mg od] also have a role in the ongoing management of these patients. The overall use of psychotropics however needs to be considered on an individual basis.

Prognosis

The prognosis of this condition is unknown, mainly because a dearth of long-term follow-up data in these patients. In a longitudinal study of 43 patients by Sneddon *et al.* [21], the authors deduced, that rather than medical intervention, it was changes in life circumstances that helped alleviate the lesions [22]. Children also appear to have a better prognosis as growing up helps them to mature and therefore manage their own problems.

CONCLUSION

Skin picking disorders and DA form a significant proportion of patients with psychiatric/psychological problems presenting with skin disease. Although the link between the skin and psyche isn't new, the lack of awareness, expertise and training make caring for this group of patients not only challenging but also results in inefficient use of resources [23]. For better outcomes, the authors propose that these patients are best managed in a dedicated psycho dermatology setting with an integrated multidisciplinary team approach.

CONFLICT OF INTEREST

The authors confirm that they have no conflict of interest to declare for this publication.

ACKNOWLEDGEMENTS

Declared none.

REFERENCES

[1] Gupta MA. Emotional regulation, dissociation, and the self-induced dermatoses: clinical features and implications for treatment with mood stabilizers. Clin Dermatol 2013; 31(1): 110-7. [http://dx.doi.org/10.1016/j.clindermatol.2011.11.015] [PMID: 23245982]

[2] Odlaug B, Grant J. Trichotillomania, Skin Picking, and Other Body-Focused Repetitive Behaviors Pathological skin picking. Washington, DC: American Psychiatric Publishing 2011; pp. 21-41.

[3] Wilhelm S, Keuthen NJ, Deckersbach T, *et al.* Self-injurious skin picking: clinical characteristics and comorbidity. J Clin Psychiatry 1999; 60(7): 454-9. [http://dx.doi.org/10.4088/JCP.v60n0707] [PMID: 10453800]

[4] Koo JY. Psychodermatology: a practical manual for clinicians. Curr Probl Dermatol 1995; (6): 204-32. [http://dx.doi.org/10.1016/S1040-0486(09)80012-4]

[5] Fruensgaard K. Psychotherapeutic strategy and neurotic excoriations. Int J Dermatol 1991; 30(3): 198-203. [http://dx.doi.org/10.1111/j.1365-4362.1991.tb03851.x] [PMID: 2037405]

[6] Fruensgaard K. Psychotherapy and neurotic excoriations. Int J Dermatol 1991; 30(4): 262-5. [http://dx.doi.org/10.1111/j.1365-4362.1991.tb04634.x] [PMID: 2050453]

[7] Gupta MA, Levenson JL. Psychiatric Care of the Medically ill The American Psychiatric Publishing Textbook of Psychosomatic Medicine. 2nd ed. American Psychiatric Publishing Inc 2011; pp. 667-90.

[8] Lee CS, Koo JY. Psychocutaneous Diseases. 2012.

[9] EDF Guidelines on the Treatment of Acne. European Dermatology Forum.

[10] Rogers M, Fairley M, Santhanam R. Artefactual skin disease in children and adolescents. Australas J Dermatol 2001; 42(4): 264-70. [http://dx.doi.org/10.1046/j.1440-0960.2001.00533.x] [PMID: 11903159]

[11] Mohandas P, Bewley A, Taylor R. Dermatitis artefacta and artefactual skin disease: the need for a psychodermatology multidisciplinary team to treat a difficult condition. Br J Dermatol 2013; 169(3): 600-6. [http://dx.doi.org/10.1111/bjd.12416] [PMID: 23646995]

[12] Gandy DT. The concept and clinical aspects of factitial dermatitis. South Med J 1953; 46(6): 551-4. [http://dx.doi.org/10.1097/00007611-195306000-00004] [PMID: 13076759]

[13] Lyell A. Cutaneous artifactual disease. A review, amplified by personal experience. J Am Acad Dermatol 1979; 1(5): 391-407.
[http://dx.doi.org/10.1016/S0190-9622(79)70032-6] [PMID: 512084]

[14] Shelley WB. Dermatitis artefacta induced in a patient by one of her multiple personalities. Br J Dermatol 1981; 105(5): 587-9.
[http://dx.doi.org/10.1111/j.1365-2133.1981.tb00804.x] [PMID: 6457622]

[15] Fabisch W. Psychiatric aspects of dermatitis artefacta. Br J Dermatol 1980; 102(1): 29-34.
[http://dx.doi.org/10.1111/j.1365-2133.1980.tb05668.x] [PMID: 7378280]

[16] Farber SK. Self-Medication, traumatic re-enactment, and somatic expressions in bulemic and self-mutilating behavior. Clin Soc Work J 1997; (25): 87-106.
[http://dx.doi.org/10.1023/A:1025785911606]

[17] Koblenzer CS. Dermatitis artefacta. Clinical features and approaches to treatment. Am J Clin Dermatol 2000; 1(1): 47-55.
[http://dx.doi.org/10.2165/00128071-200001010-00005] [PMID: 11702305]

[18] Van Moffaert M, Vermander F, Kint A. Dermatitis artefacta. Int J Dermatol 1985; 24(4): 236-8.
[http://dx.doi.org/10.1111/j.1365-4362.1985.tb05769.x] [PMID: 4008154]

[19] Jermain DM, Crismon ML. Pharmacotherapy of obsessive-compulsive disorder. Pharmacotherapy 1990; 10(3): 175-98.
[PMID: 2196535]

[20] Kawahara T, Henry L, Mostaghimi L. Needs assessment survey of psychocutaneous medicine. Int J Dermatol 2009; 48(10): 1066-70.
[http://dx.doi.org/10.1111/j.1365-4632.2009.04127.x] [PMID: 19785088]

[21] Sneddon I, Sneddon J. Self-inflicted injury: a follow-up study of 43 patients. Br Med J 1975; 30;3(5982): 527-30.
[http://dx.doi.org/10.1136/bmj.3.5982.527]

[22] Murray SJ, Ross JB, Murray AH. Life-threatening dermatitis artefacta. Cutis 1987; 39(5): 387-8.
[PMID: 3581910]

[23] Atkar R, Bewley AP, Taylor R. The cost effectiveness of a dedicated psycho-dermatology service in managing patients with dermatitis artefacta. 2012; Br J Derm 2012; 167 ((Suppl) 167): 43.

CHAPTER 6

Understanding the Challenges in Management of Delusional Infestations

Mona Malakouti[1,2] and **Jenny Murase**[2,3,*]

[1] *Chicago Medical School, Rosalind Franklin University of Medicine and Science, IL, USA*

[2] *University of California San Francisco, Department of Dermatology CA, USA*

[3] *Palo Alto Foundation Medical Group, Department of Dermatology, Mountain View, CA, USA*

Abstract: Delusional infestation (DI) is a psychodermatologic disorder characterized by the presence of a fixed, false belief that one is infested with living or non-living organisms. Patients with DI also endorse associated abnormal cutaneous symptoms such as crawling, biting or itching. DI can be extremely debilitating, as patients seek treatment and resort to self-injurious behaviors to eliminate fictional pathogens. Thus, patients may present with skin changes secondary to skin picking and excoriations. Patients with DI most often seek the help of dermatologists, because they are unable to appreciate a psychiatric etiology for their disorder; dermatologists are key to establishing both treatment and psychiatric referral for these challenging encounters. Having an informed and optimized approach in handling DI patients is vital, as clinical interactions with these patients could otherwise be unproductive and unpleasant. With good therapeutic rapport and a strong doctor-patient relationship, dermatologists may implement effective treatment with newer, second-generation anti-psychotic medications or pimozide. In this chapter, the clinical presentation, diagnostic and interpersonal approach, as well as the treatment of DI, are reviewed.

Keywords: Anti-psychotics, Delusion, Delusional infestation, Delusional parasitosis, Infestation, Parasitosis, Pimozide.

* **Corresponding author Jenny Murase:** Palo Alto Foundation Medical Group, Department of Dermatology, 701 East El Camino Real (31-104), Mountain View, CA 94040, USA; Tel: 650-934-7676; Fax: 650-934-7696; E-mail: jemurase@gmail.com.

Klas Nordlind & Anna Zalewska-Janowska (Eds.)

INTRODUCTION

Delusional infestation (DI) is a condition characterized by a fixed, false belief that one is infested with animate or inanimate matter in the absence of any objective evidence [1]. The nomenclature of this condition has changed over time to encompass the evolving definition and presentation of patients with this type of monosymptomatic delusional hypochondriasis. DI was first introduced in the late 1890s as 'acarophobie' [2, 3], and followed by similar '-phobia' ending terms, such as parasitophobia. These terms were considered to be a misnomer given that phobias are on the spectrum of an anxiety rather than delusional disorder. To reflect the delusional aspect of the disorder, delusional parasitosis or delusions of parasitosis have been preferentially used in the last half-century [4]. However, recent literature has recommended a shift of the nomenclature to delusional infestation given that patients may describe non-parasitic infesting pathogens [5, 6].

DI is a relatively well-known psychodermatologic condition that may be one of the most challenging encounters a dermatologist may face. On average, it is estimated that dermatologists will encounter two to three patients every five years, or at the very least one patient in their career [7]. DI patients are more apt to seek the help of a dermatologist rather than a psychiatrist, since they are unable to recognize an underlying psychiatric etiology for their condition. This proves difficult for dermatologists, because without insight to their disease, DI patients often reject effective antipsychotic medications and psychiatric referrals.

Even though the optimal management of these patients would also involve a psychiatrist, dermatologists may face this difficult task alone. To effectively handle these patients, an optimized approach to their care and management are of utmost importance. This chapter aims to summarize salient points regarding the clinical presentation, diagnosis, interpersonal approach, and treatment of patients with DI.

CLINICAL PRESENTATION

The classical DI patient is frequently a middle-aged to elderly woman with limited social interactions and no prior history of mental illness. Other classical cases may involve elderly men or women with comorbid dementia or other organic brain disorder, and regular recreational drugs users [8]. While there is a female predominance observed in those over the age of 50, there is an equal gender distribution in patients younger than 50 years old.

DI patients most classically endorse infestation with a parasite; however, they may also believe other living organisms, such as fungi, bacteria, worms, or other insects, are the infesting agents [9]. In addition to the infestation, patients may describe abnormal sensations such as crawling, biting, or stinging that they attribute to cutaneous pathogens in the absence of any empirical evidence substantiating their presence. The onset of DI is usually insidious and chronic in duration [10], although some patients may have episodic or transient symptoms.

A smaller subset of patients may report infestation with inanimate objects such as filaments, fibers, hairs or other particles, which is known by some as Morgellons disease [11, 12]. Since 2002, much attention has been given to Morgellons disease, with information readily available online and supported by a relatively large community of patients. Followers of Morgellons disease espouse an infectious etiology rather than a psychologic cause for this dermopathy [13]. As a provider, knowing of Morgellons can be helpful, as patients may present with a self-diagnosis of this condition having studied Internet resources.

Occasionally, patients may cohabitate with another person sharing the same delusion of infestation. This phenomenon is known as folie á deux, which can occur in 5 to 15% of cases [14, 15]. Usually one person experiences the delusion first, and induces the delusion in the other [14]. It is most often observed between husband and wife, probably owing to one attempting to show devotion and support for the other. Recovery typically involves and is dependent on treatment of both cohabitants.

DI patients can be very detailed; they may offer particulars regarding the shape, color or movement of these imaginary pathogens, along with the initiating event or perceived cause of the infestation. Frequently, patients endorse transmission from other humans, plants, infested homes and to a lesser extent animals or pets. In many cases, patients also believe their relatives to be infested. Thus, patients will often report putting forth excessive efforts in to extermination of imaginary pathogens [16 - 18], such as having repeated pesticide treatments of their homes or by applying corrosive and toxic chemicals directly to their skin. They may also obsessively launder their clothing or linen and meticulously clean their homes.

Besides going through rounds of self-treatment, patients often present having had a slew of evaluations by multiple providers including other dermatologists, infectious disease specialists or entomologists. They may mistake numerous creams or treatments, since they are usually convinced of their diagnosis of infestation and are simply looking for eradication. The may mistake or perceive negative diagnostic results by these physicians as incompetence, because they lack insight into their disease.

Specimen Sign

In preparation for their clinical visits, DI patients might present with skin samples or specimens that could include crusts, scabs, hair, skin flakes or other skin debris; this is known as the 'specimen sign' [19]. Other patients may collect specimens with adhesive tape or place them in small jars. Within the samples, there may even be colorful strings or insects; strings are often fibers from clothing, and insects may be coincidentally placed. Patients have also been recently reported to present photographs or films of sample specimens in this evolving technological age [19].

Although patients with DI classically present with skin samples as discussed above, they may not. When patients do not present with skin samples, it is useful to encourage they bring samples to their next visit to demonstrate interest, build rapport, and to create an opportunity of reviewing the slides with them [20]. To simplify collection of specimens for the patient, glass slides may be provided with special instructions to only provide what they consider to be the "best" and most relevant samples. Encouraging the use of transparent clear tape rather than matte tape is recommended to preserve the slide.

DIAGNOSTIC APPROACH

There are two types of DI, primary and secondary, thus an appropriate physical and work-up are warranted to distinguish these diagnostically [15]. The diagnosis of primary DI can be made when patients present with two of the following: a solitary belief of infestation despite the lack of microbiological evidence, and endorsement of associated abnormal cutaneous symptoms such as biting or crawling. Primary DI is considered to be a somatic subtype of delusional disorder, according to the Diagnostic and Statistical Manual of Mental Disorders, fifth edition [21]. The criteria in the DSM-V requires the delusion last longer than one month, and that the patient does not emanate bizarre, impaired thinking or hallucinations better explained by a diagnosis of schizophrenia or other mental disorder such as substance abuse, obsessive compulsive disorder or body dysmorphic disorder [21]. Although primary DI is thought to be an encapsulated or stand-alone diagnosis, a retrospective study highlighted that comorbid psychiatric diagnoses may be common in patients with DI [22, 23]. These authors suggest that an appropriate screen should be conducted for other possible comorbid psychiatric diseases for appropriate management, as they may contribute to DI symptoms.

Secondary DI is a symptom rather than a disorder, and is caused by another underlying medical or psychiatric disease. Secondary DI may occur in combination with other psychiatric disorders such as depression, anxiety, schizophrenia, obsessive-compulsive disorder, or substance abuse disorders. Medical conditions that cause secondary DI include true parasitosis, diabetes mellitus, thyroid disease, syphilis, HIV, drug side effects, hematologic disease, central nervous system disorders and nutritional insufficiencies such as vitamin B12 deficiency [10, 24 - 26]. Although cumbersome, an appropriate work-up to evaluate these possible etiologies should be considered, especially in the presence of reasonable clinical suspicion (Table **1**).

To evaluate the possibility of a true infestation, it is helpful to inquire about recent travel, and exposure to other potentially infested individuals or environments. Clinical suspicion may be heightened if patients have high peripheral eosinophilia or systemic findings corroborating infestation.

Completing a thorough physical exam will aid in properly excluding other differential diagnoses and enhance the patient's trust that a comprehensive workup is being conducted. Often, the physical exam will reveal secondary skin changes such as excoriations, ulcers, scars or secondary skin infections that have resulted from skin picking or scratching; these often present asymmetrically in areas of physical reach. Occasionally, a primary dermatologic disease that could contribute to these symptoms may be identified. Patients with transient acantholytic dermatosis or difficult-to-diagnose scabies may be mistakenly misdiagnosed with DI [27]. Upon initial presentation, patients with cutaneous dysesthesia may present with symptoms of formication, and if left untreated for a prolonged period of time, these patients may become vulnerable to believing an infestation is the cause [28]. Appropriately treating patients with cutaneous dysesthesia may prevent their progression and vulnerability to the development of DI [28]. Similarly, a recent case report described the diagnosis of peripheral neuropathy that was preceded by a diagnosis of DI prior to neurologic evaluation and nerve conduction studies in a woman complaining of formications [29].

Table (1). Appropriate work up that may be conducted for patients with possible DI to investigate secondary causes that may contribute to their presentation.

Potential Work- Up to Evaluate Possible Underlying Medical Conditions	
CBC w/diff	Albumin
Electrolytes	Serum total calcium
Urea	Phosphorus
Creatinine	Iron studies
LFTs	Serum IgE
Serum glucose	Antinuclear Antibody
TSH	Rheumatoid factor
B12	CRP/ESR
Folate	Urine analysis
Urine toxicology screen	Pregnancy test
HIV	Hepatitis C
RPR for syphilis	Cancer screening

Performing biopsies for patients with DI has been controversial. Although not always medically indicated, patients may adamantly request a biopsy hoping that an infestation or other cause will be identified [30, 31]. Some studies have indicated that the performance of a biopsy does not typically change the medical diagnosis or management of the patient, given that only secondary non-specific skin changes are usually observed by pathologic examination [32]. Besides considering diagnostic and therapeutic outcome, dermatologists could bear in mind the value a biopsy may serve in illustrating their desire to thoroughly investigate the cause of a delusional patient's symptoms. In turn, a negative biopsy may also be a valuable tool in conveying the absence of an infesting pathogen to patients [28, 33]. Moreover, denying very persistent DI patients a biopsy could be detrimental to the establishment of a potentially strong therapeutic alliance.

If the decision to perform a biopsy has been made, dermatologists should make a verbal agreement with the patient that only one biopsy will be performed [20]. It is best to allow the patient to choose the site for biopsy (reasonable location), to prevent the patient from being able to accuse the provider of picking a sub-optimal site that would explain negative results. Another agreement dermatologists could make with these patients is that if the results are in fact negative, patients will try to abandon their exhaustive search of elucidating the cause of their symptoms, and shift their focus to treatment.

The Approach to Patients with Delusional Infestations

The approach to patients with DI is two-fold. A physician's interpersonal approach and relationship with the patient can prove to be of greatest importance. Another important aspect of care is to initiate and facilitate the treatment of DI patients with effective psychodermatologic medications. Below, we will make recommendations on useful approaches to patients with DI.

Establishing a Therapeutic Alliance

Considering the patient's first clinical visit and impression may determine future interactions and the ability to build strong therapeutic rapport, the initial approach should be optimized. If a patient is referred by another provider with a potential diagnosis of DI, it is recommended that providers schedule them at the end of clinic so that more time could be devoted to their care. Providers might find it helpful to prepare for these types of encounters and to mindfully acknowledge the countless specialists and great frustration these patients will likely present with. It is important for providers to present themselves as a "fresh start" to diminish the negative ideas these patients may carry into the encounter. Also displaying a high level of positivity and enthusiasm is helpful; a neutral demeanor could make providers vulnerable to a DI patient's negative projection.

When beginning a conversation with a delusional patient, allow them to speak freely initially for a few minutes to show interest and respect for their concerns. Although with DI patients, particularly those with severely rigid delusions, a structured conversation is most helpful; providers should not be afraid of redirecting and controlling the conversation with close-ended rather than open-ended questions. This tactic prevents both the provider and patient from experiencing aggravation and distraction from the intended goal of treatment.

After identifying the patient's chief complaint, it is helpful to connect with patients by explicitly stating the patient's symptoms are "unique, complex, and mysterious" to convey interest as the provider. By communicating one's fascination and belief that the patient experiences these symptoms, they may entrust in the physician's ability and willingness to help them.

When recognizing the curiousness of the patient's symptoms, it is important to convey understanding that their described symptoms are subjectively very real, even if objectively unexplained. However, dermatologists should never confirm the possibility of an actual infestation if there is none, as this may worsen the severity and rigidity of the delusion. Providers should also avoid confronting or trying to rationally argue with patients who have DI, unless patients exhibit an overvalued idea rather than a true delusion. Alternatively, providers could relate to patients by admitting that they have seen similar phenomenon in other patients even though the cause of their symptoms has remained mostly unidentified and unexplained.

Approaching Pharmacologic Therapies For DI

Pharmacologic therapy should only be discussed once therapeutic rapport has been established. In order to facilitate and broach the topic of psychodermatologic therapies, it is helpful to explain and set realistic goals with patients who may be fixated on identifying etiology of their disease rather than being receptive to receiving treatment. Having given them a proper work up and the opportunity to view specimen slides, it is important to shift their focus to treating their symptoms even if the cause of their symptoms remain to be elucidated. To further this concept, it may be helpful to state that for medical diseases of unknown etiology, trial and error with treatments targeting symptomatic relief can be helpful.

When discussing anti-psychotic medication therapies, it is important to explicitly tell the patient that if they investigate the medication on the Internet they may see these medications are indicated for the treatment of psychotic disorders such as schizophrenia. It is helpful to tell patients that as the provider, you do not believe that they have schizophrenia and that a different dose of the medication is being used than what is typically given for schizophrenics [34].

Contrary to popular belief, once patients with DI are started on psychotropic medications for treatment of DI, they are likely to adhere [34]. In a study of 69 patients, high compliance was observed; although, some were found to discontinue for secondary reasons, many of which were preventable. Patients were found to discontinue the medication if they experienced side effects or felt the medication was ineffective. Preventable reasons for discontinuation of treatment included improper counseling and inadequate education of patients prior to initiating treatment. Thus, appropriately managing expectations of medication efficacy as well as potential side effects are both important for increasing compliance and adherence.

PHARMACOLOGIC THERAPY FOR DI

Various antipsychotic medications are available for the treatment of DI. Traditionally, pimozide has been the treatment of choice for DI; however due to its extrapyramidal side effects and potential for cardiotoxicity, some favor safer atypical antipsychotics as first line [14, 35] (Table **2**).

Most antipsychotics, both first and second generation, cause a favorable response in patients with DI [36]. If patients do not respond to one antipsychotic, changing to another is usually effective [24, 36, 37]. Besides antipsychotic medications, combination treatment with antidepressants such as selective serotonin reuptake inhibitors (SSRIs) may be useful in treating depressive symptoms associated with DI or secondary DI [8, 34, 38, 39].

Table 2. Side effect profile of antipsychotic medications that may be considered for treatment of DI.

Side Effect Profile of Selected Antipsychotic Medications for the Treatment of DI							
Agent	QTc	EPS	S	Ach	BP	MD	Prolactin
Pimozide	++	+++	+	-	+	+	++
Risperidone	+	++	+	-	++	++	+++
Olanzapine	+	+	++	++	+	+++	-
Quetiapine	++	-	++	+	++	++	-
Aripiprazole	+	+	+	-	-	-	-

Abbreviations: QTc= QTc prolongation, EPS: Extrapyramidal side effect, S: Sedation, Ach: anticholinergic effects, BP: Orthostatic hypotension, MD: Metabolic disorders Key: +++, Severe; ++, moderate; +, mild; +/-, infrequent; -, absent.

Although pimozide is a typical antipsychotic that blocks DH2 and 5HT2 receptors, it has an FDA label indication for the treatment of Tourrette syndrome, a neurologic disorder characterized by stereotyped, involuntary and repetitive tics. As a result, patients may be more accepting of treatment with pimozide, a medication typically prescribed for a neurologic disorder, rather than a safer, atypical antipsychotic medication indicated for the treatment of disorders on the spectrum of psychosis.

Pimozide should be avoided in patients with cardiac disease, the elderly, those with a history of syncope or family history of sudden death, and in combination with other QT interval prolonging medications [28]. To start pimozide, a baseline EKG should be performed due to the potential dose-dependent side effect of QT prolongation [40]. An EKG may be repeated when the patient has reached a therapeutic dose. Careful attention should be paid to patients on other medications, where there may be drug-drug interactions or additive prolongation of the QT interval [41]. The FDA has contraindicated the co-administration of pimozide with: macrolide antibiotics, azole antifungals, protease inhibitors, or zileuton [42]. Providers should also screen medications of patients with comorbid psychiatric diagnoses, since drugs like SSRIs should not be given with pimozide concomitantly, because they are thought to raise the toxicity of pimozide.

Although the side effects of pimozide are considerable, the low doses used to treat DI have not yet resulted in any reported cases of tardive dyskinesia or cardiac arrhythmias in the psychodermatologic literature [43, 44].

The dose of antipsychotic medications required to treat patients with DI is typically lower than patients with other psychotic disorders. Pimozide should be initiated at very low doses and incrementally increased, because of potential for extrapyramidal side effects and QT prolongation. Typically patients are started on a 1 mg daily dose and increased by 1 mg increments every two to three weeks until an optimal clinical response is observed or until reaching an optimally effective dose of 5 mg per day. A good clinical response is the resolution of formications rather than an absence of the delusion itself [9].

If patients experience extrapyramidal side effects such as akathisia or muscle stiffness, diphenhydramine 25 mg three times daily or benztropine 1 to 2 mg every six hours as needed may be prescribed [28, 44]. To avoid long-term tardive dyskinesia, or the development of repetitive, involuntary movements such as lip-smacking, pimozide may be tapered after patients have received an optimal dose for at least 2-3 months. The dose is tapered at a rate of 1 mg every one to four weeks. Pimozide is usually given for a total duration of 5-6 months, and may be repeated for those who experience recurrent delusions.

In more recent literature, the use of atypical antipsychotics such as risperidone [45 - 47], olanzapine [36, 48, 49] quetiapine [46], aripiprazole [50, 51], and paliperidone [8] has been addressed. Where traditional or first-generation anti-psychotics more commonly cause extrapyramidal side effects, second generation antipsychotics (SGAs) cause less. On the other hand, SGAs are more likely to cause weight gain or metabolic disorders such as hyperlipidemia and diabetes. SGAs may have less problematic drug-drug interactions, although this is independent on each individual medication. For example, combining risperidone with an SSRI is preferable to the combination of pimozide with an SSRI.

Similar to pimozide, SGAs should be initiated at low doses and slowly incrementally increased over time. These medications are also eventually tapered and discontinued after 4-6 months, although a subset of patients are more prone to relapse and require longer treatment [52]. If patients relapse, treatment may be reconstituted [44]. SGAs are also less likely to be problematic due to the lower extra-pyramidal effects if patients are treated for longer periods of time when required [53]. Although caution should be taken with giving any antipsychotic medications to the elderly, age-adjusted doses of SGAs may be considered for older patients with DI [42].

Risperidone is typically initiated at 0.5 mg twice daily, and increased in divided doses of 1 mg daily every 5 to 7 days until reaching a therapeutic dose of 3 to 6 mg daily or a maximum of 8 mg per day. Risperidone may cause rhinitis, dizziness and anxiety. It may also cause dose-dependent side effects of sedation, fatigue and QT interval prolongation. It is also important to inquire about and monitor for hyperprolactinemia with the use of risperidone, which can cause galactorrhea, increased risk of fractures, lower bone density and sexual dysfunction [52].

Olanzapine is usually started at 2.5 mg/day until reaching a range of 2.5 to 7.5 mg per day [49]. Although higher doses are used in schizophrenia, no more than 10 mg is usually necessary in DI. Olanzapine has a higher association with metabolic disturbances in glucose and lipids, as compared to other SGAs [42]. Thus, monitoring for weight gain, HbA1c, fasting glucose or lipids is recommended. Olanzapine can be more sedating, so a nighttime dose may be more appropriate.

Quetiapine is initiated at 12.5 mg every night and increased to a typical dose of 200 mg nightly [1, 42, 52]. When first beginning the medication, quetiapine's sedative effect may be more prominent, but decreases over time. Quetiapine causes less extrapyramidal side effects, but can cause QT prolongation like pimozide. Other side effects of quetiapine include orthostatic hypotension, akasthisia, dry mouth and weight gain.

Aripiprazole, a newer atypical antipsychotic, has a unique mechanism of action; it partially agonizes the D2 and 5-HT1A receptors, while it has antagonistic effects on the 5-HT2A receptor. Aripiprazole also has a better side effect profile than the first generation and other SGAs [54]. As aripiprazole blocks dopamine to a lesser extent, less extrapyramidal side effects are observed [55]. In addition, less cholesterol elevation, weight gain, hyperglycemia and hyperprolactinemia are observed with the use of aripiprazole [56]. Aripiprazole may be started at 2-5 mg daily and slowly increased by the same rate to 10-15 mg daily [44]. Aripiprazole may be stimulating and can be taken in the mornings. It is useful in patients who have poor adherence since the drug has a longer half-life, and is less likely to be affected by missed doses [57].

CONCLUSION

Patients with delusional infestation provide dermatologists with a challenging encounter. Knowing the clinical presentation of these patients, and understanding the difficulties they faced prior to their presentation is key in effectively connecting with these patients. Most of these patients have seen countless providers in search of an answer for their debilitating symptoms. Many of these patients have also undergone multiple treatments and various exterminations trying to rid themselves of these fictional pathogens. Even still, patients with DI can be greatly helped, once a good therapeutic rapport and relationship with the patient has been established. Systematically and optimally approaching these patients will assist in establishing rapport and allowing dermatologists to provide much needed treatment with effective antipsychotic medications. Newer SGAs allow for effective treatment of DI with a safer side effect profile than traditional antipsychotic medications like pimozide. Nonetheless, pimozide remains a useful, effective treatment for DI and may be used when other antipsychotic medications are ineffective.

CONFLICT OF INTEREST

The authors confirm that they have no conflict of interest to declare for this publication.

ACKNOWLEDGEMENTS

Declared none.

REFERENCES

[1] Heller MM, Wong JW, Lee ES, *et al.* Delusional infestations: clinical presentation, diagnosis and treatment. Int J Dermatol 2013; 52(7): 775-83.
[http://dx.doi.org/10.1111/ijd.12067] [PMID: 23789596]

[2] Thibierge G. Les acarophobes. J Prat Rev Gen Clin Ther 1894; 32: 373.

[3] Perrin L. Des nevrodermies parasitophobiques. Ann Dermato Syph 1896; 7: 129-38.

[4] J.W. Wilson HEM. Delusions of parasitosis (Acarophobia). Arch Dermatol Syph 1946; 54: 39.
[http://dx.doi.org/10.1001/archderm.1946.01510360043006]

[5] Freudenmann RW, Lepping P, Huber M, *et al.* Delusional infestation and the specimen sign: a European multicentre study in 148 consecutive cases. Br J Dermatol 2012; 167(2): 247-51.
[http://dx.doi.org/10.1111/j.1365-2133.2012.10995.x] [PMID: 22583072]

[6] Bewley AP, Lepping P, Freudenmann RW, Taylor R. Delusional parasitosis: time to call it delusional infestation. Br J Dermatol 2010; 163(1): 1-2.
[http://dx.doi.org/10.1111/j.1365-2133.2010.09841.x] [PMID: 20645978]

[7] Schairer D, Schairer L, Friedman A. Psychology and psychiatry in the dermatologist?(tm)s office: an approach to delusions of parasitosis. J Drugs Dermatol 2012; 11(4): 543-5.
[PMID: 22453598]

[8] Freudenmann RW, Lepping P. Delusional infestation. Clin Microbiol Rev 2009; 22(4): 690-732.
[http://dx.doi.org/10.1128/CMR.00018-09] [PMID: 19822895]

[9] Koo JY, Do JH, Lee CS. Psychodermatology. J Am Acad Dermatol 2000; 43(5 Pt 1): 848-53.
[http://dx.doi.org/10.1067/mjd.2000.109274] [PMID: 11050592]

[10] Bhatia MS, Jhanjee A, Srivastava S. Delusional infestation: a clinical profile. Asian J Psychiatr 2013; 6(2): 124-7.
[http://dx.doi.org/10.1016/j.ajp.2012.09.008] [PMID: 23466108]

[11] Robles DT, Olson JM, Combs H, Romm S, Kirby P. Morgellons disease and delusions of parasitosis. Am J Clin Dermatol 2011; 12(1): 1-6.
[http://dx.doi.org/10.2165/11533150-000000000-00000] [PMID: 21110523]

[12] Dewan P, Miller J, Musters C, Taylor RE, Bewley AP. Delusional infestation with unusual pathogens: a report of three cases. Clin Exp Dermatol 2011; 36(7): 745-8.
[http://dx.doi.org/10.1111/j.1365-2230.2011.04086.x] [PMID: 21933231]

[13] Murase JE, Wu JJ, Koo J. Morgellons disease: a rapport-enhancing term for delusions of parasitosis. J Am Acad Dermatol 2006; 55(5): 913-4.
[http://dx.doi.org/10.1016/j.jaad.2006.04.042] [PMID: 17052509]

[14] Lepping P, Freudenmann RW. Delusional parasitosis: a new pathway for diagnosis and treatment. Clin Exp Dermatol 2008; 33(2): 113-7.
[http://dx.doi.org/10.1111/j.1365-2230.2007.02635.x] [PMID: 18205853]

[15] Foster AA, Hylwa SA, Bury JE, *et al.* Delusional infestation: clinical presentation in 147 patients seen at Mayo Clinic. J Am Acad Dermatol 2012; 67(4): e1-10.

[16] Munro A. Monosymptomatic hypochondriacal psychosis manifesting as delusions of parasitosis. A description of four cases successfully treated with pimozide. Arch Dermatol 1978; 114(6): 940-3. [http://dx.doi.org/10.1001/archderm.1978.01640180074018] [PMID: 666333]

[17] Lyell A. Delusions of parasitosis. J Am Acad Dermatol 1983; 8(6): 895-7. [http://dx.doi.org/10.1016/S0190-9622(83)80024-3] [PMID: 6863652]

[18] Berrios GE. Delusional parasitosis and physical disease. Comp psychiat 1985; 26(5): 395-403.

[19] Freudenmann RW, Kolle M, Schonfeldt-Lecuona C, Dieckmann S, Harth W, Lepping P. Delusional parasitosis and the matchbox sign revisited: the international perspective. Acta Derm Venereol 2010; 90(5): 517-9. [http://dx.doi.org/10.2340/00015555-0909] [PMID: 20814630]

[20] Heller MM. KJYM Delusions of Parasitosis. Newton: Handbooks in Health Care Company 2011.

[21] Diagnostic and Statistical Manual of Mental Disorders. DSM-5. 5th ed., Arlington, VA: American Psychiatric Association 2013.

[22] Trabert W. Shared psychotic disorder in delusional parasitosis. Psychopathology 1999; 32(1): 30-4. [http://dx.doi.org/10.1159/000029063] [PMID: 9885397]

[23] Hylwa SA, Foster AA, Bury JE, Davis MD, Pittelkow MR, Bostwick JM. Delusional infestation is typically comorbid with other psychiatric diagnoses: review of 54 patients receiving psychiatric evaluation at Mayo Clinic. Psychosomatics 2012; 53(3): 258-65. [http://dx.doi.org/10.1016/j.psym.2011.11.003] [PMID: 22458994]

[24] Huber M, Lepping P, Pycha R, Karner M, Schwitzer J, Freudenmann RW. Delusional infestation: treatment outcome with antipsychotics in 17 consecutive patients (using standardized reporting criteria). Gen Hosp Psychiatry 2011; 33(6): 604-11. [http://dx.doi.org/10.1016/j.genhosppsych.2011.05.013] [PMID: 21762999]

[25] Musso MW, Jones GN, Heck MC, Gouvier D. Delusional parasitosis as a presenting feature of HIV dementia: a case study. Appl Neuropsychol Adult 2013; 20(1): 66-72. [http://dx.doi.org/10.1080/09084282.2012.704602] [PMID: 23373687]

[26] Ozten E, Tufan AE, Cerit C, Sayar GH, Ulubil IY. Delusional parasitosis with hyperthyroidism in an elderly woman: a case report. J Med Case Reports 2013; 7: 17. [http://dx.doi.org/10.1186/1752-1947-7-17] [PMID: 23305525]

[27] Bak R, Tumu P, Hui C, Kay D, Burnett J, Peng D. A review of delusions of parasitosis, part 1: presentation and diagnosis. Cutis 2008; 82(2): 123-30. [PMID: 18792544]

[28] Levin EC, Gieler U. Delusions of parasitosis. Semin Cutan Med Surg 2013; 32(2): 73-7. [http://dx.doi.org/10.12788/j.sder.0004] [PMID: 24049963]

[29] Sales PM, Thomas FP, Gondim FdeA. Delusional parasitosis heralding the diagnosis of peripheral neuropathy. Arq Neuropsiquiatr 2013; 71(2): 131-2. [http://dx.doi.org/10.1590/S0004-282X2013000200017] [PMID: 23392329]

[30] Fabbro S, Aultman JM, Mostow EN. Delusions of parasitosis: ethical and clinical considerations. J Am Acad Dermatol 2013; 69(1): 156-9.

[http://dx.doi.org/10.1016/j.jaad.2013.02.012] [PMID: 23768288]

[31] Heller MM, Murase JE, Koo JY. Practice gaps. Time and effort to establish therapeutic rapport with delusional patients: comment on ?oDelusional infestation, including delusions of parasitosis??. Arch Dermatol 2011; 147(9): 1046.
[http://dx.doi.org/10.1001/archdermatol.2011.237] [PMID: 21931042]

[32] Hylwa SA, Bury JE, Davis MD, Pittelkow M, Bostwick JM. Delusional infestation, including delusions of parasitosis: results of histologic examination of skin biopsy and patient-provided skin specimens. Arch Dermatol 2011; 147(9): 1041-5.
[http://dx.doi.org/10.1001/archdermatol.2011.114] [PMID: 21576554]

[33] Koo J, Lee CS. Delusions of parasitosis. A dermatologist?(tm)s guide to diagnosis and treatment. Am J Clin Dermatol 2001; 2(5): 285-90.
[http://dx.doi.org/10.2165/00128071-200102050-00003] [PMID: 11721647]

[34] Ahmed A, Bewley A. Delusional infestation and patient adherence to treatment: an observational study. Br J Dermatol 2013; 169(3): 607-10.
[http://dx.doi.org/10.1111/bjd.12392] [PMID: 23600661]

[35] Lepping P, Russell I, Freudenmann RW. Antipsychotic treatment of primary delusional parasitosis: systematic review. Br J Psychiatry 2007; 191: 198-205.
[http://dx.doi.org/10.1192/bjp.bp.106.029660] [PMID: 17766758]

[36] Freudenmann RW, Lepping P. Second-generation antipsychotics in primary and secondary delusional parasitosis: outcome and efficacy. J Clin Psychopharmacol 2008; 28(5): 500-8.
[http://dx.doi.org/10.1097/JCP.0b013e318185e774] [PMID: 18794644]

[37] Lepping P, Baker C, Freudenmann RW. Delusional infestation in dermatology in the UK: prevalence, treatment strategies, and feasibility of a randomized controlled trial. Clin Exp Dermatol 2010; 35(8): 841-4.
[http://dx.doi.org/10.1111/j.1365-2230.2010.03782.x] [PMID: 20184615]

[38] Delacerda A, Reichenberg JS, Magid M. Successful treatment of patients previously labeled as having ?odelusions of parasitosis?? with antidepressant therapy. J Drugs Dermatol 2012; 11(12): 1506-7.
[PMID: 23377524]

[39] Cupina D, Boulton M. Secondary delusional parasitosis treated successfully with a combination of clozapine and citalopram. Psychosomatics 2012; 53(3): 301-2.
[http://dx.doi.org/10.1016/j.psym.2011.09.005] [PMID: 22560648]

[40] Wolverton SE. Comprehensive Dermatologic Drug Therapy. 2nd ed., Philadelphia, PA: Saunders Elsevier 2007.

[41] Lorenzo CR, Koo J. SPimozide in dermatologic practice: a comprehensive review. Am J Clin Dermatol 2004; 5(5): 339-49.

[42] Sandoz A, LoPiccolo M, Kusnir D. A clinical paradigm of delusions of parasitosis. J Am Acad Dermatol 2008; 59(4): 698-704.

[43] Lee CS. Delusions of parasitosis. Dermatol Ther 2008; 21(1): 2-7.

[44] Koblenzer CS. The current management of delusional parasitosis and dermatitis artefacta. Skin Ther Lett 2010; 15(9): 1-3.

[45] De Leon OA, Furmaga KM, Canterbury AL . Risperidone in the treatment of delusions of infestation. Int J Psychiat 1997; 27(4): 403-9.

[46] Gallucci G , Beard G. Risperidone and the treatment of delusions of parasitosis in an elderly patient. Psychosomatics 1995; 36(6): 578-80.

[47] Wenning MT, Davy LE, Catalano G. Atypical antipsychotics in the treatment of delusional parasitosis. Ann Clin Psychiat 2003; 15(3-4): 233-9.

[48] Nakaya M. Olanzapine treatment of monosymptomatic hypochondriacal psychosis. Gen Hosp Psychiat 2004; 26(2): 166-7.

[49] Meehan WJ, Badreshia S, Mackley CL. Successful treatment of delusions of parasitosis with olanzapine. Arch Dermatol 2006; 142(3): 352-5.

[50] Rocha FL, Hara C. Aripiprazole in delusional parasitosis: Case report. Prog Neuro-psych 2007; 31(3): 784-6.

[51] Ladizinski B, Busse KL, Bhutani T, *et al.* Aripiprazole as a viable alternative for treating delusions of parasitosis. J Drugs Dermatol 2010; 9(12): 1531-2.

[52] Wong S, Bewley A. APatients with delusional infestation (delusional parasitosis) often require prolonged treatment as recurrence of symptoms after cessation of treatment is common: an observational study. Br J Dermatol 2011; 165(4): 893-6.

[53] Freudenmann RW, Schonfeldt-Lecuona C, Lepping P. Primary delusional parasitosis treated with olanzapine. Int Psychogeriatr 2007; 19(6): 1161-8.

[54] Bennassar A, Guilabert A, Alsina M. Treatment of delusional parasitosis with aripiprazole. Arch Dermatol 2009; 145(4): 500-1.

[55] Gupta S . Aripiprazole: Review of its pharmacology and therapeutic use in psychiatric disorders. Ann Clin Psychiat 2004; 16(3): 155-66.

[56] Kern RS GMF, Cornblatt BA, Owen JR. The neurocognitive effects of aripiprazole: an open-label comparison with olanzapine. Psychopharmacology 2006; 187(3): 312-20.

[57] Mallikaarjun S SD, Bramer SL. Pharmacokinetics, tolerability, and safety of aripiprazole following multiple oral dosing in normal healthy volunteers. J Clin Pharmacol 2004; 44: 179-87.

CHAPTER 7

Living with Psoriasis: Managing the Life Impact of Psoriasis – Practical Tips to Use in Consultation

Christine Bundy[1], **Alexandra Mizara**[2] and **Sandy R. McBride**[2,*]

[1] *The Dermatology Research Centre and Manchester Centre for Health Psychology, The University of Manchester, Manchester Academic Health Science Centre, Manchester, UK*

[2] *Department of Dermatology, Royal Free NHS Foundation Trust, London, UK*

Abstract: Psoriasis can affect every aspect of life – relationships, social life, lifestyle and work and is associated with increased levels of depression and anxiety. Understanding the beliefs, behaviours and emotions of people with psoriasis is essential to formulating effective and appropriate management plans with patients.

Psychological factors in people with psoriasis, such as alexithymia, anticipation of harm and stigma together with time constraints in clinic and skin-focused consultations, can lead to distress and life-impact going un-recognised and untreated. There is some evidence that treating distress can have a positive impact on the severity of psoriasis, and that distress in the form of worry is a major determinant of the outcome of treatment.

Screening for quality of life impact and distress in clinic using relevant questionnaires is a useful tool to identify patients in need of further support, and also provides a trigger to initiate discussion. A patient-centred consultation with setting of agendas for patient and clinician is an efficient way of targeting consultations. Questioning style in clinic is key to eliciting relevant responses which guide treatment decisions and inform treatment goals. Setting of patient-derived treatment goals and step-by-step mini-targeted approach to reaching the final goal ensures response to treatment is accompanied by improved life-impact.

Communicating measures of distress, quality of life and patient-derived treatment goals to general practitioners provides an educational tool and will raise the standard of care

* **Corresponding author Sandy R McBride:** Department of Dermatology, Royal Free NHS Foundation Trust, London NW3 2QG UK; Tel +44 2078302376; Fax +44 2078302247; E-mail: sandy.mcbride@nhs.net

Klas Nordlind & Anna Zalewska-Janowska (Eds.)

for people with psoriasis.

Keywords: Alcohol, Alexithymia, Anti-depressant, Anxiety, Beliefs, Cognitive-behaviour-therapy, Consultation, Coping, Depression, Distress, Hypnosis, Life-impact, Lifestyle, Obesity, Psoriasis, Psychology, Shame, Smoking, Stigma, Suicide.

> **"Each morning, I vacuum my bed. My torture is skin deep: there is no pain, not even itching.... Lusty, though we are loathsome to love. Keen-sighted, though we hate to look upon ourselves. The name of the disease, spiritually speaking, is Humiliation."** John Updike [1].

CASE STUDY

A 39-year-old man with psoriasis attends a dermatology clinic for the first time. He has had psoriasis since the age of 9 years. His PASI (Psoriasis Area Severity Index) score is 18.9 (severe) and his DLQI (Dermatology Life Quality Index) is 3 (minimal life-impact). The Dermatologist tells him, in her experience, it is unusual for someone with his severity of psoriasis, for it not to have a significant effect on their life. The man starts to cry. He has never been in a relationship. He has no social life. He has been in the same job since leaving school because he is too embarrassed to go to a job interview with psoriasis on his hands and face. He merely exists, as he has done for the last 30 years. He has seen several General Practitioners over the last 30 years, but his distress and the impact of his psoriasis on his life has not been recognised.

The Dermatologist who saw him in clinic was able to determine the major effect this gentleman's psoriasis was having on his life and formulate an appropriate management plan. In the consultation, she used techniques based on an understanding of psychological factors affecting people with psoriasis in order to engage the patient and identify his needs and wishes and plan his care based on managing the whole person not just his skin.

In this Chapter, we share our joint learning about people with psoriasis, and how this has changed our approach to consultations and management planning.

Illustrations are obtained from postcards distributed by the See Psoriasis: Look Deeper collaboration to people with psoriasis. The post cards were entitled 'Dear Psoriasis….' and respondents were asked to complete them either with words or images [2].

INTRODUCTION

In order to understand the full impact of psoriasis on an individual's life it is necessary to question the beliefs, emotions and behaviours of the person behind the psoriasis. Focused questioning can uncover the effect their psoriasis may have on work, relationships, social life and well-being and what is important to the patient in terms of treatment. This insight can lead to more appropriate treatment choices, improved adherence to medications and an opportunity to address the wider issues facing the individual. Communicating this understanding to patients demonstrates empathy, optimises adherence and improves satisfaction with care. Furthermore, communicating this information to the Primary Care Physician will model whole person care which can be replicated in future encounters with people with psoriasis.

PSYCHOLOGICAL FACTORS IN PSORIASIS

Key Beliefs

Beliefs and emotions drive human behaviour. Illness and treatment beliefs can explain self-management and, in particular, adherence to treatment. What people believe about (i) the disease name and associated symptoms of psoriasis make up the identity, (ii) what people believe caused psoriasis or the subsequent flares can indicate the accuracy of knowledge people have, (iii) the effects and outcome of psoriasis (consequences) indicates optimism or pessimism about living with the condition, (iv) how long they perceive the duration of psoriasis and its likely trajectory may flag up vulnerability to depression or inaccurate understanding and (v) how much they believe they, or the treatment they are receiving, can control or cure their psoriasis are particularly important signposts to likely coping strategies that may be used (see below) [3, 4].

People learn about psoriasis from a variety of sources, some helpful and accurate, and others that give partial or incorrect understanding. This collection of beliefs we term their 'personal model'. An individual's personal model has an effect on how they feel about and self-manage psoriasis. For example, if someone believes their psoriasis is caused by a food allergy there will be every reason to keep looking for the one ingredient that may be responsible for triggering their psoriasis, but no incentive to use prescribed medicines. Many patients spend large sums of money and take unknown preparations in pursuit of a cause or cure for their psoriasis based on their beliefs. This 'mindset' can affect attitudes to treatment – if someone doesn't believe a suggested medical treatment is going to work for them, they are less like to adhere to the recommended treatment regime and it is therefore less likely to be effective. Furthermore, this thinking can lead to a sense of hopelessness and helplessness, which are precursors to depression [5, 6], and excessive worrying.

Emotions

Alexithymia and Internalisation of Emotion

Some people with psoriasis find it difficult to identify and express their emotions and may even lack appropriate language to describe their emotions [7]. This is called alexithymia and can make it very difficult for friends, relations, partners and clinicians to ascertain what a person with psoriasis is actually feeling. Richards *et al.* [8] found one in three patients with psoriasis to experience alexithymia. Knowing that patients with psoriasis may experience alexithymia influences the type of questions we use in consultations. Common questions such as:

> 'How are you feeling?' or 'how have you been?'

are often used as social greetings and can be difficult to answer for someone with psoriasis alexithymia and often result in an uninformative response such as:

> 'Fine' or 'not too bad'.

Specific and more direct questions such as:

'How is your psoriasis affecting your life?'

are more likely to trigger an illuminating and helpful response in the clinical context.

People with psoriasis often internalise their emotions [9], which can cause increased stress, distress and anger [10]. The result of this internalisation can be social isolation, even within relationships, and precipitates unhelpful coping strategies such as self-medicating, over-use of alcohol and over eating in order to manage emotional issues [11]. Importantly, the emotional build up due to ineffective emotional processing can lead to worsening of psoriasis and psychological problems [12].

Stigma and Shame

Psoriasis is stigmatising. Psoriasis often attracts negative attention, public rejection and reactions of disgust [6, 13]. People with psoriasis report feeling flawed as individuals, they anticipate rejection, can be over-sensitive to other's attitudes, and feel guilt and shame. It is worth taking a moment to think just how painful these emotions are. Over 78% of people with psoriasis have experienced high levels of stigmatisation [14]. Stigmatising experiences are common. Ginsburg *et al.* [13] found 99 of 100 patients described experiencing stigmatising events and Gupta *et al.* [15] reported 26% of patients had experienced public rejection such as being asked to leave a swimming pool. Unless experienced it is difficult to imagine how it must feel to brave going to a swimming pool, putting on a swimming costume, approaching the pool and then being asked to leave in front of people, because the lifeguard thinks you have a contagious disease. Recently, Sampogna *et al.* [16] found 37% of patients experienced humiliation often or all the time, and shame was one of the most frequently reported emotions.

Unsurprisingly feelings of shame and stigma lead people to hide psoriasis and avoid sporting activities, social opportunities, intimacy and public places [17]. Patients with psoriasis develop hyper-vigilance for threat (looking for negative cues of observation linked to their psoriasis) [9, 18]. Access to health care may also be affected if people are reluctant to expose their skin even to a doctor and find it difficult to ask for help [13]. Many are not assertive enough to insist on receiving effective appropriate treatment for themselves [3]. They may not put themselves forward for life-opportunities such as work promotions and dating [19]. Awareness that patients with psoriasis may not be proactive in seeking more effective care is essential to ensuring treatments are stepped up appropriately and patients are receiving optimal management. Accurate assessment and monitoring of disease activity with validated scoring systems such as Psoriasis Area Severity Index (PASI) [20] or the Simplified Psoriasis Index (SPI) [21] is important and often identifies patients who are being under-treated.

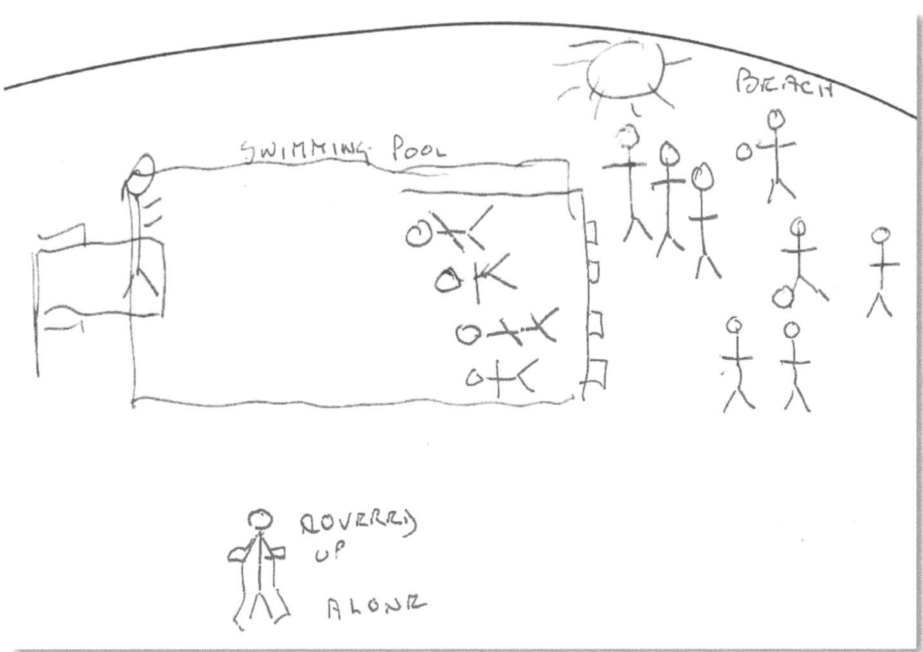

Fig. (1). Person with psoriasis depicted 'covered up alone' whilst the rest of society are playing ball and swimming in the sun [2].

Anticipation of Failure and Harm

People with psoriasis are constantly alert to negative cues or observations linked to their psoriasis [9, 18] which results in physiological over arousal. This may be a consequence of anticipating something bad is going to happen or that they will be a failure. One person with psoriasis described expecting to find his house on fire every time he drove home. This fear of failure can also explain avoidant behaviours in people with psoriasis – such as avoiding situations in which they believe they will be unsuccessful. Conversely, evidence suggests a sense of hope is associated with physical and material well-being, satisfying relationships and psychological well-being [22].

In consultations it is important to be aware that patients often don't expect to get better, or feel that treatments won't work for them (even if they are told they are effective for most other people). Despite the many effective treatments for psoriasis some people have never been told they can get better. Realistic optimism about treatment efficacy with regular reinforcement, combined with appropriate information about time-courses of treatments, are key to managing expectations, maintaining patient engagement with treatment and supporting self-efficacy beliefs about self-management of psoriasis.

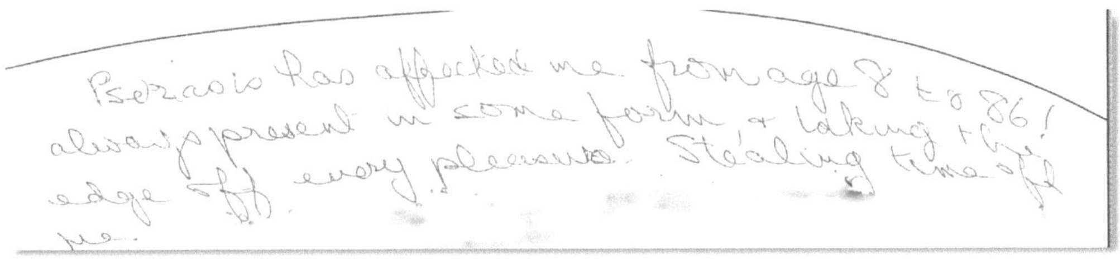

Fig. (2). Psoriasis is a long-term condition which can affect every aspect of life [2].

Behavioural Responses

Illness Coping Strategies

Coping strategies play a key role in how a long-term illness may affect an individual's life. Psoriasis is increasingly recognised as a long-term condition and there is emerging evidence for the importance of coping strategies and beliefs about psoriasis (see above) in outcomes. There is a large literature on individual coping and how this affects outcomes from long-term conditions. Although the literature is not always clear on which are the most effective strategies. Long-term as opposed to short-term or crisis management coping strategies are particularly important to adopt [23]. Short term coping strategies such as avoidance of social events may alleviate immediate distress, but lead to social isolation or increased sense of shame in the long-term.

Life Impact of Psoriasis

Psoriasis is not usually physically likely to stop people leading the lives they wish to, however, the combination of stigma, shame, attitudes of others and avoidant behaviour can result in people living very different lives to those they would have lived without psoriasis. This is well documented by Kimball *et al.* [19] in their paper on the Cumulative Life Impact of Psoriasis. People with psoriasis gradually move away from how their lives would have been without psoriasis, as they make decisions to *e.g.* not go for a job promotion, not take a relationship forward *etc.*

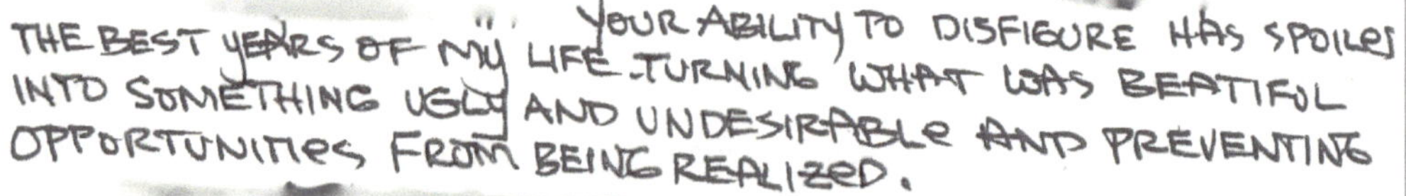

Fig. (3). Psoriasis can affect life opportunities [2].

JUDGES
With all the practice I've had. I could hoover for Britain!

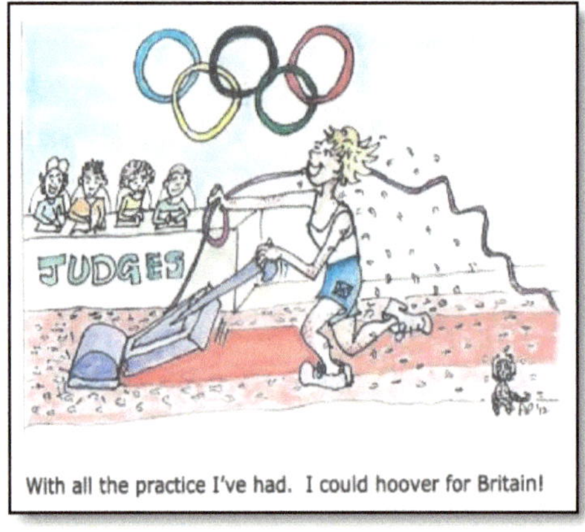

Fig. (4). Psoriasis is messy and lead to an increased burden of housework [2].

Physical Impact of Psoriasis

Psoriasis is messy! Increased skin shedding leads to daily, or several times daily vacuuming and increased dusting. Flaking and bleeding of skin onto clothing and bedding requires extra washing. Topical treatments are also messy, greasy and sometimes stain clothes, again leading to extra laundering. People with psoriasis describe not wanting to visit friends with dark coloured sofas for fear of leaving an obvious trail of skin and of taking a dustpan and brush and their own sheets on holiday or when visiting family, so as not to leave a mess. Some people with psoriasis avoid going to stay with family and friends at all due to their psoriasis.

Psoriasis is itchy (contrary to established teaching), uncomfortable and sometimes painful. It can disrupt sleep and the chronic inflammatory process may lead to fatigue. Concomitant psoriasis co-morbidities such as psoriatic arthritis, Crohn's disease and increased risk of diabetes and cardio-vascular disease (CVD) may also add to the physical impact of having psoriasis.

CLOTHES SHOP
I wish I could wear a dress but my legs are covered in psoriasis & I am too embarrassed. They are so ugly to look at

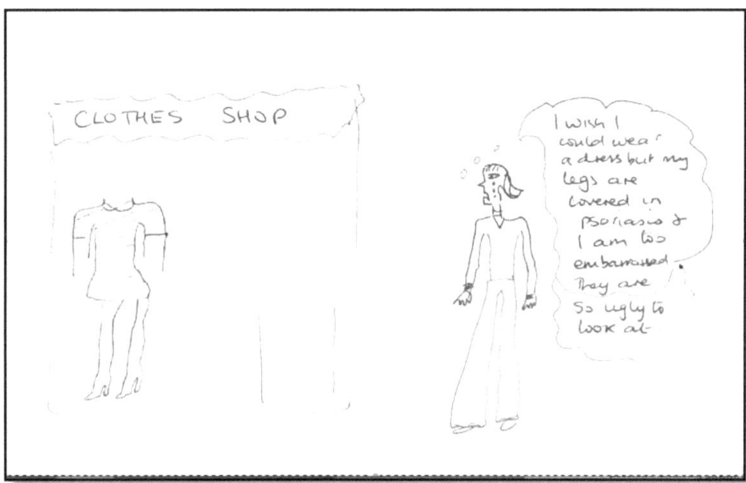

Fig. (5). Psoriasis affects the clothes people can wear [2].

Clothing

Patients with psoriasis often report not being able to wear the clothes they wish to and this bothers them. In the summer they cover up whilst people without psoriasis wear shorts and t-shirts. They also frequently wear light colours so the flakes of skin are less noticeable on their clothes. Although this may not be considered an important part of medical management, for the patient it is just another way they experience being different and leading an impoverished life with psoriasis. Asking about this directly can help reduce the stigma as patients realise they are not experiencing this alone.

Relationships

Psoriasis unsurprisingly affects relationships, with increased rates of divorce [24] and deterioration of close relationships [25]. It can also affect the choice of partner with some people choosing a partner predominantly because they are accepting of their psoriasis.

Eghlileb *et al.* [25] interviewed family members of patients with psoriasis, 57% described psychological distress, 55% social disruption, 44% limitations to leisure activities and 37% deterioration of close relationships. The patient's level of distress was more closely related to the family member's level of distress and social disruption than the severity of their psoriasis. In a multi-centre, case controlled study Poot *et al.* found severe family dysfunction to be 16 times more likely in patients with psoriasis than families without the skin condition [26].

Psoriasis can affect sexual functioning. In Gupta & Gupta's cross-sectional survey of 120 in-patients [27], 40% reported a decline in sexual activity since the onset of psoriasis. This decline was associated with joint pains, but not psoriasis severity. Sampogna *et al.* [28] confirmed impaired sexual life activity in 936 inpatients, using individual questions relating to sexual functioning from dermatology and psoriasis specific questionnaires, they found 35 - 71% of patients reported sexual problems. In contrast to Gupta and Gupta, psoriasis severity and psychological problems were associated with sexual functioning. In neither study was the presence of genital lesions determined, so the confounding effect of psoriasis affecting the genital area could not be determined.

In a cross-sectional study of 92 male patients with psoriasis, Goulding *et al.* [29] reported an increased prevalence of erectile dysfunction (ED) (58%), compared with controls with other skin conditions (49%). However, Psoriasis was not an independent risk factor for ED, atherosclerosis was thought to mediate the link between psoriasis and ED.

Difficulties in relationships are unsurprising in a condition associated with high levels of distress and stigma. Despite this, questions about the quality of relationships and sexual functioning are not routinely included in consultations or as outcomes of studies.

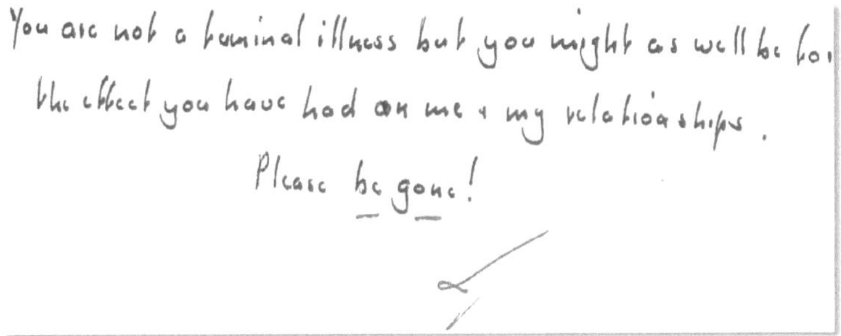

Fig. (6). Psoriasis affects relationships [2].

Social

Although psoriasis is mainly thought to be an adult-onset condition up to 30% of psoriasis originates in childhood [30]. The impact of having a disfiguring skin condition during formative years appears to be considerable. Several people who responded to the See Psoriasis: Look Deeper postcard study recalled adverse childhood experiences, despite having lived for several decades with psoriasis [2].

WHY DID GIRLS
SHUN ME LIKE I HAD THE PLAGUE, WHY
WAS I BORN, JUST TO HAVE SUCH A
LONELY EXISTENCE. WHY, WHY, WHY.

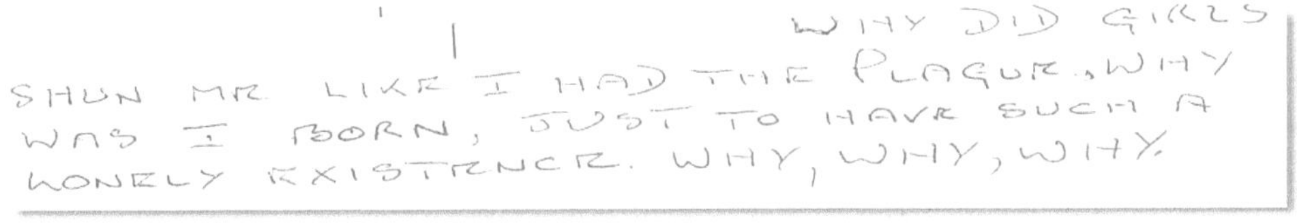

Fig. (7). Childhood psoriasis can have a profound effect [2].

Psoriasis can affect everyday experiences such as haircutting and limit social exposure and opportunities to exercise and participate in sports. This latter point could have particular repercussions for later health.

Employment and Financial Burden

As illustrated in our case-study, an individual's choice of employment or career, and therefore income, can be affected by psoriasis [31 - 33]. In one study [25] 40% of patients reported experiencing major difficulties at work, and in another [31], 2% stopped work completely due to psoriasis. There is an inverse relationship between psoriasis severity, employment and income [32 - 34] – the worse the psoriasis, the lower the income. This clearly has a cost to society with loss of productivity [35].

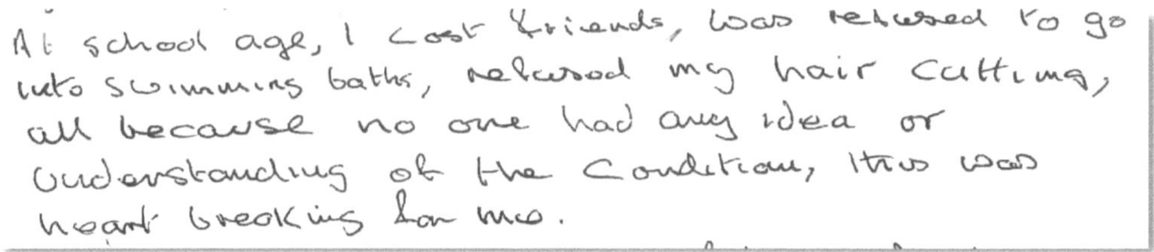

At school age, I lost friends, was refused to go
into swimming baths, refused my hair cutting,
all because no one had any idea or
understanding of the condition, this was
heart breaking for me.

Fig. (8). Psoriasis affects everyday experiences [2].

Attending for treatment can also impact on work – attending for phototherapy 3 x weekly for 8 weeks is unlikely to be compatible with work for most people. Consequently, in a hostile economic climate, taking time off work to attend for treatment makes it more likely that patients will lose their job.

Recently, biological intervention studies have incorporated broader 'life impairment' outcomes into their study designs. Psoriasis-related work productivity and activity impairment (WPAI) is significantly improved by treatment with adalimumab [34]. Treatment with ustekinumab is linked with improvement in productivity, and reduced absenteeism [33]. Both studies show strong correlations between disease severity and work disability. Kimball and colleagues [34] reported a reduction in Dermatology Life Quality Index (DLQI) was more highly correlated with WPAI outcomes than improvement in PASI score and Reich *et al.* [33] reported a greater improvement in WPAI outcomes in patients with higher DLQI scores and distress (Hospital Anxiety and Depression Score -HADS) scores at baseline, suggesting that reduction in work disability may only be partially attributable to improvement in disease severity.

Lifestyle Issues – Alcohol, Smoking and Obesity

<u>Smoking and Alcohol</u>

Excess alcohol use and cigarette smoking is common among patients with psoriasis [36, 37], Kirby *et al.* [38] reported excess alcohol consumption to be up to 50% and Mills *et al.* [39] found twice as many patients with psoriasis smoked compared to controls. Alcohol exacerbates psoriasis severity and pruritus, and can impair treatment response [40]. Poikolainen *et al.* [41] demonstrated the risk of death from alcohol-related causes was higher than expected in people with psoriasis. Naldi *et al.* [42, 43] found a trend of increased risk of psoriasis for cigarette and alcohol users. Patients often cite using smoking and alcohol in order to relieve stress but paradoxically smoking increases anxiety and dependency on external methods of control whereas well-being is enhanced with a sense of having control of one's life. Alcohol does have anxiolytic properties, particularly for social anxiety but often increases avoidant behaviours rather than promoting helpful coping

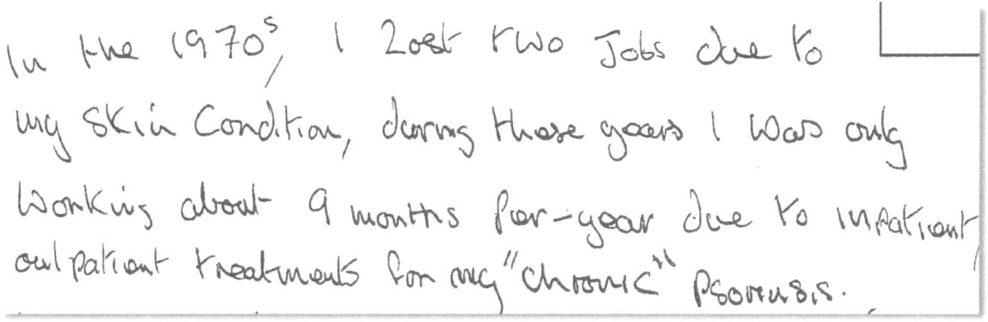
In the 1970s, I lost two jobs due to my skin condition, during those years I was only working about 9 months per-year due to inpatient/outpatient treatments for my "chronic" psoriasis.

Fig. (9). Psoriasis and treatments for psoriasis can affect employment [2].

Obesity

Obesity is also a particular issue for people with psoriasis. Raised body mass index (BMI) is associated with increased severity of psoriasis [44] and is also linked to lack of response to fixed dose medications [45]. Visceral fat is associated with pro-inflammatory immune mediators such as resistin and leptin and cytokines such as interleukin (IL)-6 and tumour necrosis factor-alpha (TNF-α) [46], hence abdominal adiposity is likely to be metabolically active and may drive psoriasis. Over-eating resulting in obesity may represent an un-helpful coping response to having psoriasis.

Restricted energy or weight reduction programmes with and without exercise for people with psoriasis can facilitate clearance of psoriasis [47 - 50] and potentially reduce CVD risk. However, many weight loss studies show short –term benefits only and the onus is on the dermatology community to design interventions that are both effective and sustainable.

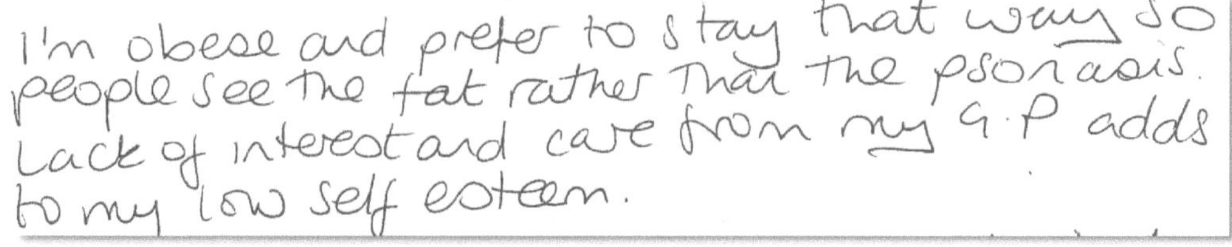

Fig. (10). Obesity is associated with psoriasis [2].

STRESS AND DISTRESS IN PSORIASIS

Stress and Psoriasis

The relationship between stress (the response to a threat we feel we can't deal with), distress (anxiety and depression) and psoriasis is well documented. Sixty percent of people describe their psoriasis as being worsened by stress [51]. Stress has been demonstrated to exacerbate psoriasis and having psoriasis can be stressful hence a spiral of events may be triggered [52]. For some people stressful situations are made worse by the fear that the stress experienced will trigger a flare of psoriasis. Stress, in the form of worry, was the major determinant of outcome of phototherapy treatment in a study by Fortune *et al.* [53]. For a more detailed review of the mechanisms of stress and psoriasis see the review article by Kleyn and colleagues [54].

Distress and Psoriasis

High levels of anxiety and depression are experienced by people with psoriasis, with estimates of between 17-30% of patients experiencing clinical depression [17, 55]. Anticipation of failure and harm, is particularly associated with anxiety and depression [9]. High rates of thoughts of suicide are reported with one study of outpatients with psoriasis 9.7% reporting a wish to be dead and 5.5% reported suicidal ideation [40]. In the UK it is estimated that 10,400 diagnoses of depression, 7,100 diagnoses of anxiety and 350 cases of suicidality are attributable to psoriasis annually [56].

One in five people with severe psoriasis are taking anti-depressant medication [57].

Interestingly, as with psoriasis, the inflammatory cytokine TNF -α may be implicated in depression [58]. There is emerging evidence to suggest that inflammatory processes in the skin may also lead to up-regulation of inflammatory markers in the brain which could lead to mood changes [59]. It is yet to be determined whether treatment with immune-modulating agents has an effect on mood, independent of the beneficial effect on severity of psoriasis.

Quite simply this is how you make me feel psoriasis. Every day.

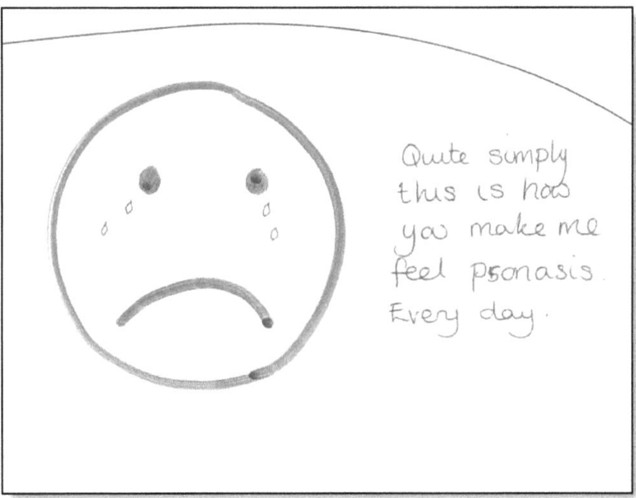

Fig. (11). Psoriasis is associated with anxiety and depression [2].

Does Treating Distress Improve Psoriasis?

Evidence regarding the effectiveness of treating distress in people with psoriasis is minimal compared with evidence about the prevalence of distress. A recent meta-analysis of psychological interventions designed to improve skin condition outcomes identified only 8 studies involving psoriasis that fulfilled criteria of having a control group, being published in a peer reviewed journal and written in English [60]. The majority of these studies had methodological flaws including small sample sizes and non-randomised study designs. A diverse range of psychological interventions with differing outcomes were included in this review, making comparisons difficult.

The main treatment modalities can be divided into psychotropic medication, cognitive-based interventions and arousal reduction techniques (treatment of physical symptoms without changing thought processing).

Psychotropic Medications

Few studies have investigated the role of psychotropic medication in psoriasis. Treatment with the monoamine oxidase inhibitor antidepressant moclobemide, in addition to topical steroid for the psoriasis was found superior compared with topical steroid alone in terms of improvement in PASI, depression and anxiety scores. However, baseline PASI scores were low (<5) in each group making it difficult to evaluate changes in scores [61]. A recent retrospective open study of 38 patients with moderate/severe psoriasis and depressive and/or anxiety disorders recently starting anti-TNFα therapy compared treatment with escitalopram (serotonin selective reuptake inhibitor) plus psychotherapeutic support with psychotherapeutic support alone [62]. Reduced depression, anxiety, pruritus and PASI scores were seen in the escitalopram plus psychotherapeutic support group compared with psychotherapeutic support only. No details of the content of 'psychotherapeutic support' were given and randomisation was by patient preference.

The evidence for psychotropic medication and psoriasis is equivocal with several case-reports of fluoxetine-induced or exacerbated psoriasis [63 - 65] and the atypical antidepressant bupropion has also been linked to exacerbations of psoriasis [66]. The mood stabiliser lithium commonly precipitates or aggravates psoriasis [67].

Psychological Interventions

Arousal Reduction

Mindfulness based stress reduction (MBSR) improved the rate of psoriasis clearance during phototherapy despite a non-significant reduction in stress [68]. A small study also confirmed twenty weeks of meditation was effective in improving psoriasis severity ($p \leq 0.01$) but psychological outcomes were not evaluated [69].

An emotional disclosure (ED) programme where people with psoriasis were asked to spend 20 minutes writing or talking about their thoughts or the most upsetting times of their lives on 4 consecutive days only resulted in an improvement in psoriasis if there was an improvement in mood [70]. Paradisi *et al.* [71] investigated the efficacy of 2 different written-emotional-disclosure techniques performed on 3 consecutive days and compared to a control group in patients just undergoing phototherapy. The results were difficult to interpret, but appear to demonstrate a slightly longer duration of remission in one of the ED groups. Both of these studies had a very short duration of intervention. The inclusion of better designed ED techniques on a more regular basis may be worth further investigation.

Hypnosis

A potential role for hypnosis has been demonstrated in two studies [72, 73]. Tausk & Whitmore [72] randomised highly or moderately hypnotisable patients with psoriasis to either hypnosis with active suggestions of improvement or just hypnosis alone. No difference in PASI scores was found between the 2 groups, although there was a suggestion that highly hypnotisable patients in both groups demonstrated a greater percentage reduction in PASI score than moderately hypnotisable patients ($p=0.01$). Participant numbers, however, were very low and there was no control group. Price *et al.* [73] employed self-hypnosis, together with relaxation and support group discussions over 8 weekly sessions in a matched controlled trial. A significant reduction in anxiety and neuroticism (tendency to emotional lability and experience emotional distress) as measured by the Eysenck personality questionnaire – revised (EPQ-R) and increase in self-esteem, maintained at 6 months, were demonstrated. However, no significant improvement in psoriasis severity was found. Both studies were limited by small group size and the improvement seen in the study by Price *et al.* cannot be attributed to self-hypnosis training alone. Hypnosis may, however, be a therapeutic modality that warrants further testing.

Cognitive Behaviour Therapy

Individual coping strategies, illness perceptions, beliefs about control and curability of illness, and individual personality traits are closely linked with health outcomes and psychological distress in psoriasis [3, 74 - 77].

Only two studies have investigated face-to face cognitive behaviour therapy (CBT) as an adjunctive treatment for psoriasis. A high quality, case-controlled study by Fortune *et al.* [78] involving 40 patients with psoriasis receiving adjunctive group CBT demonstrated a significant reduction in PASI scores at 6 weeks and 6 months follow-up, with 64% achieving >75% psoriasis clearance at 6 months follow-up compared with 23% of the control group. The CBT group also showed reductions in anxiety and depression scores and almost double the reduction in self-reported disability and life stress scores at 6 weeks and 6 months follow-up.

In a randomised controlled trial, Zacharie *et al.* [79] compared the effect of seven individual psychotherapy sessions which included imagery, stress management and relaxation training over a 12-week period with a control group in 51 patients with psoriasis. Small, but significant, reductions in specific psoriasis plaques and a non-significant trend for overall reduction in psoriasis severity were observed. Patient reported stress remained unchanged. This study was the only one to combine arousal reduction with a cognitive based intervention.

Bundy *et al.* [80] investigated the effect of a web-based tailored CBT intervention targeted at people with psoriasis. This did show a small, but statistically significant improvement in anxiety and quality of life, but not PASI score or depression scores. Baseline levels however were low and there was a lot of missing data due to a high proportion of patients leaving the study. It would be interesting to determine the effect of this web-based intervention in a patient population with high baseline scores. Furthermore, while some patients clearly benefit from CBT it is important to recognise that web-based psychological interventions may not be acceptable to many patients.

Further studies investigating the effectiveness of CBT, which include work related and relationship outcomes are also needed.

Recognition of Distress by Clinicians

Despite the high prevalence of distress in people with psoriasis, clinicians in general are not good at recognising distress in their patients and often have different treatment priorities to their patients. In a checklist completed by both dermatologists and patients [81], patients ranked "embarrassment over one's appearance" as the most severe important feature of psoriasis, whereas dermatologists ranked it the lowest. Patient (not clinician) rated severity is the strongest predictor of quality of life impairment [82 - 84]. In a study at a well-established specialist psoriasis centre, Dermatologists identified and discussed distress in just over a third (39%) only of all distressed patients. There was poor correlation between patient and clinician regarding the presence of anxiety and depression [84].

'My counselling changed my life and my vision of life. I felt suicidal and I now feel grateful for my life'

Fig. (12). Quote from a patient with psoriasis who completed a course of CBT.

Discrepancy between patients and clinicians is complex. Patients' own underlying illness beliefs, coping strategies [84 - 86], personality traits [9] and feelings of shame contribute to distress and are factors often not explored by clinicians. People with psoriasis may be reluctant to ask for help and to disclose personal information through fear of rejection and previous experiences of lack of empathy from clinicians [16, 87]. Clinicians are often under considerable time pressure in clinic and feel that asking about distress will be very time-consuming. They may also fear they won't be able to deal with the information they receive, or simply believe that it is not their job to explore the issue of distress in their patient [88, 89].

Approaching the Life Impact of Psoriasis in Clinic

The life-impact of psoriasis can be considerable, difficult to identify and troublesome to manage in the typical clinical setting. Very few Dermatology departments have the benefit of a dedicated psychology service and there are significant time-constraints in clinic [90]. Based on our experience and the evidence presented above, we suggest an approach that will help with identifying distress, providing patient-centred treatment and improving the life-impact of psoriasis for your patients and others.

Assessment of Quality of Life impact and Distress in Clinic

In order to maximise consultation time and efficiency, we suggest all patients with psoriasis complete screening questionnaires whilst waiting to see the clinician. We presently use the Dermatology Life Quality Index (DLQI) [91] to assess quality of life and the Hospital and Anxiety Depression Score (HADS) [92] to assess distress, but there are other measures available. The UK 2012 National Institute for Clinical Excellence (NICE) guidance for psoriasis [93] recommends that all patients with psoriasis are assessed for 'the impact of disease on physical, psychological and social wellbeing' but do not identify specific assessment tools. Skindex – 29 has been demonstrated to correlate better with severity of psoriasis than some other outcome measures [94]. For a comprehensive review of patient reported outcome measures for psoriasis see Kitchen *et al.* [95].

The results of the DLQI and HADS questionnaires will give a good idea as to how distressed a patient is and some idea as to the life-impact of their psoriasis, before the consultation. Used in conjunction with the PASI scoring system [20] - discrepancy in scores between clinical severity and impact of psoriasis can be identified. High impact sites such as hands, scalps and genitals are poorly represented by the PASI scoring system and involvement of these sites may be the cause of high DLQI scores with a low PASI score. Newer scoring systems such as the Simplified Psoriasis Index [21] address some of the limitations of the PASI system, but is a relatively new measure and is yet be incorporated into standard clinical practice. It is, however, included as a secondary outcome measure in some recent biologic trials. As our case study illustrated, some patients who are highly affected by their psoriasis may tick the 'not relevant' box on the DLQI questionnaire when asked if their psoriasis affects (*e.g.*) their sexual functioning or social life, if they have no sex or social life due to their psoriasis. This would give a discrepantly low DLQI score compared with PASI score in a patient who is highly affected by their psoriasis and can be identified by the clinician interpreting the DLQI sheet.

Addressing Distress

Screening questionnaires to identify distress provide an opening for discussions with patients. It is important once distress is identified that it is not ignored, as this will only exacerbate negative feelings.

Opening statements could include:

'I see you're feeling very low – how much of that is due to your psoriasis? or 'It looks like your psoriasis is having a big effect on your life'.

Often, with people with psoriasis, the responses to these questions and statements will be relatively short as they tend to internalise their emotions and are not used to discussing emotion.

Clinicians often say they are fearful of discussing patients' distress with them in case they open 'a can of worms' that they cannot manage. This suggests clinicians believe they have to be able to fix patient problems - they don't. Patients often report feeling relieved that the clinician is taking their distress seriously and asking about it conveys empathy and respect, which are important characteristics in the patient centred consultation. Engaging with a patient on an emotional level will also contribute to a trusting patient-clinician relationship, identify key areas of importance for the patient and optimise adherence to treatment.

Suggestions to discuss with a patient who is experiencing distress are:

Treating psoriasis medically and see if they feel better about their skin, re-screen at next visit and if there is no change discuss further help as below.

Ask the patients' General Practitioner (GP) to refer to their local psychology service.

Provide access to approved 'self-help' resources (see British Association of Dermatologists website for a list of approved resources).

Refer to a psychology-based psycho-dermatology service if available.

In cases of severe depression with suicide risk contact liaison psychiatrist and or clinical psychology urgently.

How to Identify Suicide Risk

Although the following questions may seem difficult to ask and clinicians may be concerned that they are suggesting suicidality, actually this is not likely and to someone who is considering suicide the questions will be perfectly acceptable and often provide evidence to people feeling suicidal that someone understands how low they feel. To someone who isn't suicidal they will be appreciative of your concern.

> 'I see you are feeling very low – how much are you troubled by thoughts of ending your life?'
>
> 'Have you thought of ways you might do this?'
>
> 'Have you made any preparations?'
>
> 'Is there anyone you are close to who you can talk to about it?'

Having identified someone who is at risk of suicide – the emergency mental health service will need to be alerted and plans made to help the individual.

Patient Centred Consultation

Since we know that there is a discrepancy between what the patient thinks is important about their psoriasis and what the clinician thinks, it is worthwhile developing a shared agenda for the consultation. Patient-centred does not mean only the patient's agenda is important. Asking at the beginning of the consultation what the patient hopes to achieve in the appointment targets the available time around what the patient wants rather than the clinician, but also allows the clinician to communicate what he/she thinks is important clinically. Other useful targeting and time-saving information questions are 'are there any treatments you're particularly interested in or any that you'd like to avoid?'

Setting goals

Setting patient-centred goals provides an opportunity to focus on how psoriasis is affecting the patient's life and which specific areas are important to them to be cleared. Useful questions to illicit illuminating answers are:

'How would your life be different if you didn't have psoriasis?'

'What would you like to do, that you're not doing now, if you didn't have psoriasis?'

'If I had a magic wand that clears psoriasis, what would you like me to do with it (you're not allowed to say 'clear my whole body')?'

It is important to document the goals and also to work out a step-by-step mini-targeted approach to reaching the final goal.

Help patients to set small achievable goals within an achievable timescale and not be over-ambitious. Check progress in relation to these goals on each visit and be prepared to revisit and re-set unachievable goals.

e.g.

Target – to wear shorts

Step 1. Buy some shorts that do not feel too revealing and wear them around the house

Step 2. Wear shorts outside walking around the block for 10 mins

Step 3. Gradually increase the amount of time wearing shorts outside

Step 4. Wear shorts all day and gradually build up the amount of skin exposure time.

At the end of the consultation:

Go through the treatment goals with the patient and the agreed treatment plan. By verbalising what the patient has told you that they are most concerned about and what they wish to address, you will provide empathy and optimise the chances of them remembering and therefore adhering to treatment. End with an action by reminding the patient what they agreed they were going to do when they leave the consultation.

Arrange a follow-up appointment to assess response to treatment (including DLQI and HADS) and discuss progress towards achieving the patient-centred goals.

Always ask if there's anything you've missed, or anything else they wanted to discuss.

This provides true value over time and, counter-intuitively, adds little extra time to the conventional consultation.

CONCLUSION

The standard skin focused consultation does not make it easy for people to talk about how psoriasis is affecting their lives. In addition, people with psoriasis often find it difficult to express and talk about emotions, feel stigmatized, are concerned about what others are thinking and think that they will fail at activities and treatment opportunities.

Patient-centred consultation styles, with patient derived goal-setting and step by step action planning towards goals is an efficient, effective way to work with treatment plans.

Communication of patient goals and the impact of psoriasis on psychological, social and physical well-being with GPs provides an educational opportunity and conveys the importance of recognising and managing psoriasis as a long-term systemic inflammatory condition.

We believe the approach to people with psoriasis described in this chapter will allow patients with psoriasis to experience timely, appropriate referral and empathic, efficient and effective patient-centred care.

CONFLICT OF INTEREST

Alexandra Mizara has no conflict of interest.

Sandy McBride has performed sponsored lectures for Lilly, Janssen, Amgen and Abbvie. She has performed consultancy work for Abbvie and is a member of the

See Psoriasis: Look Deeper collaboration, sponsored by Abbvie.

Christine Bundy has given sponsored presentations for Abbvie, Janssen, Sanofi, holds a Pfizer i-CRP research grant and is a member of the See Psoriasis: Look Deeper collaboration, sponsored by Abbvie.

ACKNOWLEDGEMENTS

Declared none.

REFERENCES

[1] J U From the Journal of a Leper. Problems and Other Stories. Fawcett Books 1972; pp. 202-18.

[2] Bundy C, Borthwick M, McAteer H, *et al.* Psoriasis: snapshots of the unspoken: using novel methods to explore patients' personal models of psoriasis and the impact on well-being. Br J Dermatol 2014; 171(4): 825-31.
[http://dx.doi.org/10.1111/bjd.13101] [PMID: 24814298]

[3] Scharloo M, Kaptein AA, Weinman J, Bergman W, Vermeer BJ, Rooijmans HG. Patients' illness perceptions and coping as predictors of functional status in psoriasis: a 1-year follow-up. Br J Dermatol 2000; 142(5): 899-907.
[http://dx.doi.org/10.1046/j.1365-2133.2000.03469.x] [PMID: 10809846]

[4] Scharloo M, Kaptein AA, Weinman J, *et al.* Illness perceptions, coping and functioning in patients with rheumatoid arthritis, chronic obstructive pulmonary disease and psoriasis. J Psychosom Res 1998; 44(5): 573-85.
[http://dx.doi.org/10.1016/S0022-3999(97)00254-7] [PMID: 9623878]

[5] Koo J. Population-based epidemiologic study of psoriasis with emphasis on quality of life assessment. Dermatol Clin 1996; 14(3): 485-96.
[http://dx.doi.org/10.1016/S0733-8635(05)70376-4] [PMID: 8818558]

[6] Kleyn CE, McKie S, Ross AR, *et al.* Diminished neural and cognitive responses to facial expressions of disgust in patients with psoriasis: a functional magnetic resonance imaging study. J Invest Dermatol 2009; 129(11): 2613-9.
[http://dx.doi.org/10.1038/jid.2009.152] [PMID: 19710691]

[7] Taylor GJ, Bagby RM, Parker JD. Disorders of affect regulation: alexithymia in medical and psychiatric illness. Cambridge, New York: Cambridge University Press 1997.
[http://dx.doi.org/10.1017/CBO9780511526831]

[8] Richards HL, Fortune DG, Griffiths CE, Main CJ. Alexithymia in patients with psoriasis: clinical correlates and psychometric properties of the Toronto Alexithymia Scale-20. J Psychosom Res 2005; 58(1): 89-96.
[http://dx.doi.org/10.1016/j.jpsychores.2004.03.009] [PMID: 15771875]

[9] Mizara A, Papadopoulos L, McBride SR. Core beliefs and psychological distress in patients with psoriasis and atopic eczema attending secondary care: the role of schemas in chronic skin disease. Br J

Dermatol 2012; 166(5): 986-93.
[http://dx.doi.org/10.1111/j.1365-2133.2011.10799.x] [PMID: 22211355]

[10] Niemeier V, Fritz J, Kupfer J, Gieler U. Aggressive verbal behaviour as a function of experimentally induced anger in persons with psoriasis. Eur J Dermatol 1999; 9(7): 555-8.
[PMID: 10523736]

[11] Schaaf H, Eipp C, Deubner R, Hesse G, Vasa R, Gieler U. [Psychosocial aspects of coping with tinnitus and psoriasis patients. A comparative study of suicidal tendencies, anxiety and depression]. HNO 2009; 57(1): 57-63. [Psychosocial aspects of coping with tinnitus and psoriasis patients. A comparative study of suicidal tendencies, anxiety and depression].
[http://dx.doi.org/10.1007/s00106-008-1800-4] [PMID: 19096811]

[12] Lumley MA. Alexithymia, emotional disclosure, and health: a program of research. J Pers 2004; 72(6): 1271-300.
[http://dx.doi.org/10.1111/j.1467-6494.2004.00297.x] [PMID: 15509283]

[13] Ginsburg IH, Link BG. Psychosocial consequences of rejection and stigma feelings in psoriasis patients. Int J Dermatol 1993; 32(8): 587-91.
[http://dx.doi.org/10.1111/j.1365-4362.1993.tb05031.x] [PMID: 8407075]

[14] Hrehorów E, Salomon J, Matusiak L, Reich A, Szepietowski JC. Patients with psoriasis feel stigmatized. Acta Derm Venereol 2012; 92(1): 67-72.
[http://dx.doi.org/10.2340/00015555-1193] [PMID: 21879243]

[15] Gupta MA, Gupta AK, Watteel GN. Perceived deprivation of social touch in psoriasis is associated with greater psychologic morbidity: an index of the stigma experience in dermatologic disorders. Cutis 1998; 61(6): 339-42.
[PMID: 9640555]

[16] Sampogna F, Tabolli S, Abeni D. Living with psoriasis: prevalence of shame, anger, worry, and problems in daily activities and social life. Acta Derm Venereol 2012; 92(3): 299-303.
[http://dx.doi.org/10.2340/00015555-1273] [PMID: 22678565]

[17] Weiss SC, Kimball AB, Liewehr DJ, Blauvelt A, Turner ML, Emanuel EJ. Quantifying the harmful effect of psoriasis on health-related quality of life. J Am Acad Dermatol 2002; 47(4): 512-8.
[http://dx.doi.org/10.1067/mjd.2002.122755] [PMID: 12271293]

[18] Fortune DG, Richards HL, Corrin A, Taylor RJ, Griffiths CE, Main CJ. Attentional bias for psoriasis-specific and psychosocial threat in patients with psoriasis. J Behav Med 2003; 26(3): 211-24.
[http://dx.doi.org/10.1023/A:1023408503807] [PMID: 12845935]

[19] Kimball AB, Gieler U, Linder D, Sampogna F, Warren RB, Augustin M. Psoriasis: is the impairment to a patient's life cumulative? J Eur Acad Dermatol Venereol 2010; 24(9): 989-1004.
[PMID: 20477920]

[20] Fredriksson T, Pettersson U. Severe psoriasis--oral therapy with a new retinoid. Dermatologica 1978; 157(4): 238-44.
[http://dx.doi.org/10.1159/000250839] [PMID: 357213]

[21] Chularojanamontri L, Griffiths CE, Chalmers RJ. The Simplified Psoriasis Index (SPI): a practical tool for assessing psoriasis. J Invest Dermatol 2013; 133(8): 1956-62.

[http://dx.doi.org/10.1038/jid.2013.138] [PMID: 23807685]

[22] Szramka-Pawlak B, Hornowska E, Walkowiak H, Zaba R. Hope as a Psychological Factor Affecting Quality of Life in Patients With Psoriasis. Appl Res Qual Life 2014; 9: 273-83. [http://dx.doi.org/10.1007/s11482-013-9222-1] [PMID: 24834136]

[23] McCrae RR. Age differences and changes in the use of coping mechanisms. J Gerontol 1989; 44(6): 161-9. [http://dx.doi.org/10.1093/geronj/44.6.P161] [PMID: 2809108]

[24] Frangos JE, Kimball AB. Divorce / marriage ratio in patients with psoriasis compared to patients with other chronic medical conditions. J Invest Dermatol 2008; 128 (Suppl. 1): S87.

[25] Eghlileb AM, Davies EE, Finlay AY. Psoriasis has a major secondary impact on the lives of family members and partners. Br J Dermatol 2007; 156(6): 1245-50. [http://dx.doi.org/10.1111/j.1365-2133.2007.07881.x] [PMID: 17459044]

[26] Poot F, Antoine E, Gravellier M, *et al.* A case-control study on family dysfunction in patients with alopecia areata, psoriasis and atopic dermatitis. Acta Derm Venereol 2011; 91(4): 415-21. [http://dx.doi.org/10.2340/00015555-1074] [PMID: 21336474]

[27] Gupta MA, Gupta AK. Psoriasis and sex: a study of moderately to severely affected patients. Int J Dermatol 1997; 36(4): 259-62. [http://dx.doi.org/10.1046/j.1365-4362.1997.00032.x] [PMID: 9169321]

[28] Sampogna F, Gisondi P, Tabolli S, Abeni D. Impairment of sexual life in patients with psoriasis. Dermatology (Basel) 2007; 214(2): 144-50. [http://dx.doi.org/10.1159/000098574] [PMID: 17341864]

[29] Goulding JM, Price CL, Defty CL, Hulangamuwa CS, Bader E, Ahmed I. Erectile dysfunction in patients with psoriasis: increased prevalence, an unmet need, and a chance to intervene. Br J Dermatol 2011; 164(1): 103-9. [http://dx.doi.org/10.1111/j.1365-2133.2010.10077.x] [PMID: 20874856]

[30] Mahé E, Maccari F, Beauchet A, *et al.* Childhood-onset psoriasis: association with future cardiovascular and metabolic comorbidities. Br J Dermatol 2013; 169(4): 889-95. [http://dx.doi.org/10.1111/bjd.12441] [PMID: 23937622]

[31] Fowler JF, Duh MS, Rovba L, *et al.* The impact of psoriasis on health care costs and patient work loss. J Am Acad Dermatol 2008; 59(5): 772-80. [http://dx.doi.org/10.1016/j.jaad.2008.06.043] [PMID: 19119095]

[32] Horn EJ, Fox KM, Patel V, Chiou CF, Dann F, Lebwohl M. Association of patient-reported psoriasis severity with income and employment. J Am Acad Dermatol 2007; 57(6): 963-71. [http://dx.doi.org/10.1016/j.jaad.2007.07.023] [PMID: 17761358]

[33] Reich K, Schenkel B, Zhao N, *et al.* Ustekinumab decreases work limitations, improves work productivity, and reduces work days missed in patients with moderate-to-severe psoriasis: results from PHOENIX 2. J Dermatolog Treat 2011; 22(6): 337-47. [http://dx.doi.org/10.3109/09546634.2010.499931] [PMID: 21034290]

[34] Kimball AB, Yu AP, Signorovitch J, *et al.* The effects of adalimumab treatment and psoriasis severity on self-reported work productivity and activity impairment for patients with moderate to severe

psoriasis. J Am Acad Dermatol 2012; 66(2): e67-76.
[http://dx.doi.org/10.1016/j.jaad.2010.10.020] [PMID: 21616560]

[35] Sohn S, Schoeffski O, Prinz J, *et al.* Cost of moderate to severe plaque psoriasis in Germany: a multicenter cost-of-illness study. Dermatology (Basel) 2006; 212(2): 137-44.
[http://dx.doi.org/10.1159/000090654] [PMID: 16484820]

[36] Higgins EM, Peters TJ, du Vivier AW. Smoking, drinking and psoriasis. Br J Dermatol 1993; 129(6): 749-50.
[http://dx.doi.org/10.1111/j.1365-2133.1993.tb03349.x] [PMID: 8286268]

[37] McAleer MA, Mason DL, Cunningham S, *et al.* Alcohol misuse in patients with psoriasis: identification and relationship to disease severity and psychological distress. Br J Dermatol 2011; 164(6): 1256-61.
[http://dx.doi.org/10.1111/j.1365-2133.2011.10345.x] [PMID: 21457207]

[38] Kirby B, Richards HL, Mason DL, Fortune DG, Main CJ, Griffiths CE. Alcohol consumption and psychological distress in patients with psoriasis. Br J Dermatol 2008; 158(1): 138-40.
[PMID: 17999698]

[39] Mills CM, Srivastava ED, Harvey IM, *et al.* Smoking habits in psoriasis: a case control study. Br J Dermatol 1992; 127(1): 18-21.
[http://dx.doi.org/10.1111/j.1365-2133.1992.tb14818.x] [PMID: 1637689]

[40] Gupta MA, Schork NJ, Gupta AK, Kirkby S, Ellis CN. Suicidal ideation in psoriasis. Int J Dermatol 1993; 32(3): 188-90.
[http://dx.doi.org/10.1111/j.1365-4362.1993.tb02790.x] [PMID: 8444530]

[41] Poikolainen K, Karvonen J, Pukkala E. Excess mortality related to alcohol and smoking among hospital-treated patients with psoriasis. Arch Dermatol 1999; 135(12): 1490-3.
[http://dx.doi.org/10.1001/archderm.135.12.1490] [PMID: 10606054]

[42] Naldi L, Parazzini F, Brevi A, *et al.* Family history, smoking habits, alcohol consumption and risk of psoriasis. Br J Dermatol 1992; 127(3): 212-7.
[http://dx.doi.org/10.1111/j.1365-2133.1992.tb00116.x] [PMID: 1390163]

[43] Naldi L. Cigarette smoking and psoriasis. Clin Dermatol 1998; 16(5): 571-4.
[http://dx.doi.org/10.1016/S0738-081X(98)00040-6] [PMID: 9787967]

[44] Tobin AM, Hackett CB, Rogers S, *et al.* Body mass index, waist circumference and HOMA-IR correlate with the Psoriasis Area and Severity Index in patients with psoriasis receiving phototherapy. Br J Dermatol 2014; 171(2): 436-8.
[http://dx.doi.org/10.1111/bjd.12914] [PMID: 24641699]

[45] Mease PJ, Goffe BS, Metz J, VanderStoep A, Finck B, Burge DJ. Etanercept in the treatment of psoriatic arthritis and psoriasis: a randomised trial. Lancet 2000; 356(9227): 385-90.
[http://dx.doi.org/10.1016/S0140-6736(00)02530-7] [PMID: 10972371]

[46] Jensen MD. Role of body fat distribution and the metabolic complications of obesity. J Clin Endocrinol Metab 2008; 93(11) (Suppl. 1): S57-63.
[http://dx.doi.org/10.1210/jc.2008-1585] [PMID: 18987271]

[47] Farias MM, Achurra P, Boza C, Vega A, de la Cruz C. Psoriasis following bariatric surgery: clinical

evolution and impact on quality of life on 10 patients. Obes Surg 2012; 22(6): 877-80. [http://dx.doi.org/10.1007/s11695-012-0646-8] [PMID: 22488682]

[48] Hossler EW, Wood GC, Still CD, Mowad CM, Maroon MS. The effect of weight loss surgery on the severity of psoriasis. Br J Dermatol 2013; 168(3): 660-1. [letter]. [http://dx.doi.org/10.1111/j.1365-2133.2012.11211.x] [PMID: 22880618]

[49] Jensen P, Zachariae C, Christensen R, *et al.* Effect of weight loss on the severity of psoriasis: a randomized clinical study. JAMA Dermatol 2013; 149(7): 795-801. [http://dx.doi.org/10.1001/jamadermatol.2013.722] [PMID: 23752669]

[50] Naldi L, Conti A, Cazzaniga S, *et al.* Diet and physical exercise in psoriasis: a randomized controlled trial. Br J Dermatol 2014; 170(3): 634-42. [http://dx.doi.org/10.1111/bjd.12735] [PMID: 24641585]

[51] Fortune DG, Richards HL, Main CJ, Griffiths CE. What patients with psoriasis believe about their condition. J Am Acad Dermatol 1998; 39(2 Pt 1): 196-201. [http://dx.doi.org/10.1016/S0190-9622(98)70074-X] [PMID: 9704828]

[52] Verhoeven EW, Kraaimaat FW, Jong EM, Schalkwijk J, van de Kerkhof PC, Evers AW. Effect of daily stressors on psoriasis: a prospective study. J Invest Dermatol 2009; 129(8): 2075-7. [letter]. [http://dx.doi.org/10.1038/jid.2008.460] [PMID: 19194471]

[53] Fortune DG, Richards HL, Kirby B, *et al.* Psychological distress impairs clearance of psoriasis in patients treated with photochemotherapy. Arch Dermatol 2003; 139(6): 752-6. [http://dx.doi.org/10.1001/archderm.139.6.752] [PMID: 12810506]

[54] Hunter HJ, Griffiths CE, Kleyn CE. Does psychosocial stress play a role in the exacerbation of psoriasis? Br J Dermatol 2013; 169(5): 965-74. [http://dx.doi.org/10.1111/bjd.12478] [PMID: 23796214]

[55] Lynde CW, Poulin Y, Guenther L, Jackson C. The burden of psoriasis in Canada: insights from the pSoriasis Knowledge IN Canada (SKIN) survey. J Cutan Med Surg 2009; 13(5): 235-52. [http://dx.doi.org/10.2310/7750.2009.08071] [PMID: 19769832]

[56] Kurd SK, Troxel AB, Crits-Christoph P, Gelfand JM. The risk of depression, anxiety, and suicidality in patients with psoriasis: a population-based cohort study. Arch Dermatol 2010; 146(8): 891-5. [PMID: 20713823]

[57] Meyer N, Paul C, Feneron D, *et al.* Psoriasis: an epidemiological evaluation of disease burden in 590 patients. J Eur Acad Dermatol Venereol 2010; 24(9): 1075-82. [PMID: 20236205]

[58] Postal M, Appenzeller S. The importance of cytokines and autoantibodies in depression. Autoimmun Rev 2015; 14(1): 30-5. [http://dx.doi.org/10.1016/j.autrev.2014.09.001] [PMID: 25242344]

[59] Miller AH, Maletic V, Raison CL. Inflammation and its discontents: the role of cytokines in the pathophysiology of major depression. Biol Psychiatry 2009; 65(9): 732-41. [http://dx.doi.org/10.1016/j.biopsych.2008.11.029] [PMID: 19150053]

[60] Lavda AC, Webb TL, Thompson AR. A meta-analysis of the effectiveness of psychological interventions for adults with skin conditions. Br J Dermatol 2012; 167(5): 970-9.

[http://dx.doi.org/10.1111/j.1365-2133.2012.11183.x] [PMID: 22924999]

[61] Alpsoy E, Ozcan E, Cetin L, *et al.* Is the efficacy of topical corticosteroid therapy for psoriasis vulgaris enhanced by concurrent moclobemide therapy? A double-blind, placebo-controlled study. J Am Acad Dermatol 1998; 38(2 Pt 1): 197-200.
[http://dx.doi.org/10.1016/S0190-9622(98)70240-3] [PMID: 9486674]

[62] D'Erme AM, Zanieri F, Campolmi E, *et al.* Therapeutic implications of adding the psychotropic drug escitalopram in the treatment of patients suffering from moderate-severe psoriasis and psychiatric comorbidity: a retrospective study. J Eur Acad Dermatol Venereol 2014; 28(2): 246-9.
[http://dx.doi.org/10.1111/j.1468-3083.2012.04690.x] [PMID: 22963277]

[63] Hemlock C, Rosenthal JS, Winston A. Fluoxetine-induced psoriasis. Ann Pharmacother 1992; 26(2): 211-2.
[PMID: 1554934]

[64] Tan Pei Lin L, Kwek SK. Onset of psoriasis during therapy with fluoxetine. Gen Hosp Psychiatry 2010; 32(4): 446.e9-446.e10.
[http://dx.doi.org/10.1016/j.genhosppsych.2009.08.008] [PMID: 20633754]

[65] Tamer E, Gur G, Polat M, Alli N. Flare-up of pustular psoriasis with fluoxetine: possibility of a serotoninergic influence? J Dermatolog Treat 2009; 20(3): 1-3.
[http://dx.doi.org/10.1080/09546630802449096] [PMID: 18850415]

[66] Cox NH, Gordon PM, Dodd H. Generalized pustular and erythrodermic psoriasis associated with bupropion treatment. Br J Dermatol 2002; 146(6): 1061-3.
[http://dx.doi.org/10.1046/j.1365-2133.2002.04679.x] [PMID: 12072078]

[67] Basavaraj KH, Ashok NM, Rashmi R, Praveen TK. The role of drugs in the induction and/or exacerbation of psoriasis. Int J Dermatol 2010; 49(12): 1351-61.
[http://dx.doi.org/10.1111/j.1365-4632.2010.04570.x] [PMID: 21091671]

[68] Kabat-Zinn J, Wheeler E, Light T, *et al.* Influence of a mindfulness meditation-based stress reduction intervention on rates of skin clearing in patients with moderate to severe psoriasis undergoing phototherapy (UVB) and photochemotherapy (PUVA). Psychosom Med 1998; 60(5): 625-32.
[http://dx.doi.org/10.1097/00006842-199809000-00020] [PMID: 9773769]

[69] Gaston L, Lassonde M, Bernier-Buzzanga J, Hodgins S, Crombez JC. Psoriasis and stress: a prospective study. J Am Acad Dermatol 1987; 17(1): 82-6.
[http://dx.doi.org/10.1016/S0190-9622(87)70176-5] [PMID: 3611457]

[70] Vedhara K, Morris RM, Booth R, Horgan M, Lawrence M, Birchall N. Changes in mood predict disease activity and quality of life in patients with psoriasis following emotional disclosure. J Psychosom Res 2007; 62(6): 611-9.
[http://dx.doi.org/10.1016/j.jpsychores.2006.12.017] [PMID: 17540218]

[71] Paradisi A, Abeni D, Finore E, *et al.* Effect of written emotional disclosure interventions in persons with psoriasis undergoing narrow band ultraviolet B phototherapy. Eur J Dermatol 2010; 20(5): 599-605.
[PMID: 20605769]

[72] Tausk F, Whitmore SE. A pilot study of hypnosis in the treatment of patients with psoriasis.

Psychother Psychosom 1999; 68(4): 221-5.
[http://dx.doi.org/10.1159/000012336] [PMID: 10396014]

[73] Price ML, Mottahedin I, Mayo PR. Can psychotherapy help patients with psoriasis? Clin Exp Dermatol 1991; 16(2): 114-7.
[http://dx.doi.org/10.1111/j.1365-2230.1991.tb00319.x] [PMID: 2032371]

[74] Richards HL, Fortune DG, Griffiths CE. Adherence to treatment in patients with psoriasis. J Eur Acad Dermatol Venereol 2006; 20(4): 370-9.
[http://dx.doi.org/10.1111/j.1468-3083.2006.01565.x] [PMID: 16643132]

[75] Rapp SR, Cottrell CA, Leary MR. Social coping strategies associated with quality of life decrements among psoriasis patients. Br J Dermatol 2001; 145(4): 610-6.
[http://dx.doi.org/10.1046/j.1365-2133.2001.04444.x] [PMID: 11703288]

[76] Wahl AK, Robinson HS, Langeland E, Larsen MH, Krogstad AL, Moum T. Clinical characteristics associated with illness perception in psoriasis. Acta Derm Venereol 2014; 94(3): 271-5.
[http://dx.doi.org/10.2340/00015555-1673] [PMID: 24002676]

[77] Wahl A, Hanestad BR, Wiklund I, Moum T. Coping and quality of life in patients with psoriasis. Qual Life Res 1999; 8(5): 427-33.
[http://dx.doi.org/10.1023/A:1008944108101] [PMID: 10474284]

[78] Fortune DG, Richards HL, Kirby B, Bowcock S, Main CJ, Griffiths CE. A cognitive-behavioural symptom management programme as an adjunct in psoriasis therapy. Br J Dermatol 2002; 146(3): 458-65.
[http://dx.doi.org/10.1046/j.1365-2133.2002.04622.x] [PMID: 11952546]

[79] Zachariae R, Oster H, Bjerring P, Kragballe K. Effects of psychologic intervention on psoriasis: a preliminary report. J Am Acad Dermatol 1996; 34(6): 1008-15.
[http://dx.doi.org/10.1016/S0190-9622(96)90280-7] [PMID: 8647966]

[80] Bundy C, Pinder B, Bucci S, Reeves D, Griffiths CE, Tarrier N. A novel, web-based, psychological intervention for people with psoriasis: the electronic Targeted Intervention for Psoriasis (eTIPs) study. Br J Dermatol 2013; 169(2): 329-36.
[http://dx.doi.org/10.1111/bjd.12350] [PMID: 23551271]

[81] Baughman RD, Sobel R. Psoriasis. A measure of severity. Arch Dermatol 1970; 101(4): 390-5.
[http://dx.doi.org/10.1001/archderm.1970.04000040012004] [PMID: 5440812]

[82] Sampogna F, Johansson V, Axtelius B, Abeni D, Söderfeldt B. Quality of life in patients with dental conditions: comparing patients' and providers' evaluation. Community Dent Health 2009; 26(4): 234-8.
[PMID: 20088222]

[83] Choi J, Koo JY. Quality of life issues in psoriasis. J Am Acad Dermatol 2003; 49(2) (Suppl.): S57-61.
[http://dx.doi.org/10.1016/S0190-9622(03)01136-8] [PMID: 12894127]

[84] Richards HL, Fortune DG, Weidmann A, Sweeney SK, Griffiths CE. Detection of psychological distress in patients with psoriasis: low consensus between dermatologist and patient. Br J Dermatol 2004; 151(6): 1227-33.
[http://dx.doi.org/10.1111/j.1365-2133.2004.06221.x] [PMID: 15606519]

[85] Fortune DG, Richards HL, Main CJ, Griffiths CE. Patients' strategies for coping with psoriasis. Clin Exp Dermatol 2002; 27(3): 177-84.
[http://dx.doi.org/10.1046/j.1365-2230.2002.01055.x] [PMID: 12072002]

[86] Richards HL, Fortune DG, Chong SL, *et al.* Divergent beliefs about psoriasis are associated with increased psychological distress. J Invest Dermatol 2004; 123(1): 49-56.
[http://dx.doi.org/10.1111/j.0022-202X.2004.22703.x] [PMID: 15191541]

[87] Fortune DG, Richards HL, Griffiths CE, Main CJ. Psychological stress, distress and disability in patients with psoriasis: consensus and variation in the contribution of illness perceptions, coping and alexithymia. Br J Clin Psychol 2002; 41(Pt 2): 157-74.
[http://dx.doi.org/10.1348/014466502163949] [PMID: 12034003]

[88] Nelson PA, Keyworth C, Chisholm A, *et al.* 'In someone's clinic but not in mine'--clinicians' views of supporting lifestyle behaviour change in patients with psoriasis: a qualitative interview study. Br J Dermatol 2014; 171(5): 1116-22.
[http://dx.doi.org/10.1111/bjd.13231] [PMID: 24981809]

[89] C W Understanding skin problems: acne, eczema, psoriais and related conditions. NJ: Wiley 2003.

[90] Bewley A, Burrage DM, Ersser SJ, Hansen M, Ward C. Identifying individual psychosocial and adherence support needs in patients with psoriasis: a multinational two-stage qualitative and quantitative study. J Eur Acad Dermatol Venereol 2014; 28(6): 763-70.
[http://dx.doi.org/10.1111/jdv.12174] [PMID: 23663069]

[91] Lewis V, Finlay AY. 10 years experience of the Dermatology Life Quality Index (DLQI). J Investig Dermatol Symp Proc 2004; 9(2): 169-80.
[http://dx.doi.org/10.1111/j.1087-0024.2004.09113.x] [PMID: 15083785]

[92] Zigmond AS, Snaith RP. The hospital anxiety and depression scale. Acta Psychiatr Scand 1983; 67(6): 361-70.
[http://dx.doi.org/10.1111/j.1600-0447.1983.tb09716.x] [PMID: 6880820]

[93] Psoriasis C S. The assessment and management of psoriasis. NICE guidelines [CG153] 2012.

[94] Fernandez-Peñas P, Jones-Caballero M, Espallardo O, García-Díez A. Comparison of Skindex-29, Dermatology Life Quality Index, Psoriasis Disability Index and Medical Outcome Study Short Form 36 in patients with mild to severe psoriasis. Br J Dermatol 2012; 166(4): 884-7.
[http://dx.doi.org/10.1111/j.1365-2133.2012.10806.x] [PMID: 22229951]

[95] Kitchen H, Cordingley L, Young H, Griffiths CE, Bundy C. Patient-reported outcome measures in psoriasis: the good, the bad and the missing! Br J Dermatol 2015; 172(5): 1210-21.
[http://dx.doi.org/10.1111/bjd.13691] [PMID: 25677764]

CHAPTER 8

Psychological Treatments for Dermatological Conditions

Andrea W.M. Evers*, **Saskia Spillekom-van Koulil** and **Sylvia van Beugen**

Leiden University, Institute of Psychology, Health, Medical and Neuropsychology Unit, Faculty of Social and Behavioral Science, Leiden, and Radboud University Medical Centre, Department of Medical Psychology, Nijmegen, The Netherlands

Abstract: The impact of dermatological conditions on a patient's life is frequently underestimated. Patients with skin conditions experience several physical complaints, including itch, pain and fatigue. Furthermore, in comparison to the general population, patients report a decreased psychological well-being, lowered quality of life and feelings of stigmatization and shame. Psychological treatments are widely used in addition to regular dermatological treatments to improve physical and psychological functioning of patients with chronic skin conditions. These treatments are usually aimed at changing the psychosocial factors that can influence the onset and/or course of skin conditions, such as dysfunctional coping behaviors, itch-scratching problems and stress. There are unimodal interventions in which single treatments are used, for example psychoeducation or relaxation exercises, and multimodal treatments in which a variety of different interventions are applied based on cognitive-behavioral therapy and self-management principles. Furthermore, a distinction can be made between interventions that focus primarily on skin-related psychosocial problems, interventions that focus on itch-scratching problems, and interventions that are focused on psychiatric problems in the dermatological practice. This chapter gives an overview on the psychosocial factors relevant for dermatological conditions, relevant diagnostic methods and the content and scientific evidence of specific psychological treatments in these different categories.

* **Corresponding author Andrea W.M. Evers:** University of Leiden, Institute of Psychology, Health, Medical and Neuropsychology Unit, Faculty of Social Science, PO Box 9555 / 2300 RB Leiden / The Netherlands; Tel: +31-71-527 6891; Fax: +31-71-527 3619; E-mail: a.evers@fsw.leidenuniv.nl.

Klas Nordlind & Anna Zalewska-Janowska (Eds.)

Keywords: Cognitive-behavioral therapy, Dermatological conditions, Habit reversal, Itch-scratching problems, Psychological treatment, Stress management.

INTRODUCTION

The impact of skin conditions on a patient's everyday life is frequently underestimated. Although the influence of psychological factors on the skin has been recognized since a long time, systematic research on psychological factors and treatments has only begun in the last decades. Research shows that people with skin conditions experience more physical symptoms, such as itch, pain and fatigue than the general population [1]. Patients additionally report more anxiety, tension and depressive feelings, and experience social restrictions [2 - 4]. Psychological treatments have consequently been regularly proposed as possible added benefit for the regular dermatological treatments. Based on the existing research evidence focusing particularly on highly prevalent chronic skin conditions, this chapter focuses on the psychosocial factors relevant for dermatological conditions and their impact on daily life, relevant diagnostic methods and psychological treatments.

PREVALENT PROBLEMS IN PATIENTS WITH DERMATOLOGICAL CONDITIONS

Skin conditions are generally characterized by their fluctuating course and they are often accompanied with physical complaints such as itch, desquamation or pain. Research shows that chronic skin conditions, such as psoriasis and eczema, are accompanied by physical, emotional and social problems and can lead to multiple restrictions in everyday life [5]. Patients report decreased psychological well-being and lower quality of life compared to the general population [3, 6, 7]. For 20 to 40 percent of this group, symptoms are so severe that they are considered a risk group for long-term adjustment problems which require further treatment [4]. The decreased psychosocial well-being can in turn negatively affect the skin condition; for example, patients with psoriasis who also have a high level of psychological distress benefit less from treatments such as phototherapy [8].

Patients with chronic skin conditions often state that 'itch is worse than pain'. Accordingly, itch is the most prominent complaint in most skin conditions. More than half of the patients with chronic skin conditions report to be experiencing symptoms of itch [1, 9]. The definition of itch, 'an unpleasant sensation provoking the desire to scratch', implies the strong correlation between itch and scratching. Frequent scratching can however lead to skin damage which can in turn aggravate skin conditions [9]. In many patients, scratching leads to relief in the short-term, while feelings of helplessness, shame and guilt play a big role in the long-term. Reactions from the environment towards the scratching behavior ('Could you please stop scratching yourself') can increase these feelings and cause irritation and tensions. Many patients especially suffer from itch at night, leading to sleep problems, chronic fatigue, concentration problems and increased irritability during the day. Over time this can lead to increased avoidance of everyday activities and in the longer term to depressive moods [3]. Accordingly, patients with chronic itch report lower psychological and social well-being than the general population [2 - 4]. Besides itch, skin conditions can also be accompanied by pain [1], for example in patients with chronic ulcera. In addition, eczemas or open wounds caused by scratching can also cause painful fissures in the skin.

Patients with chronic skin conditions additionally report more restrictions in social activities, work and leisure than the general population. Multiple factors can play a role in this. Medical treatments of skin conditions are often quite time intensive, for example when an ointment has to be applied to the whole body several times a day. Additionally patients report feeling restricted by the effect of ointments on their clothes and by the smell of certain ointments such as coal tar ointments. Due to the visibility of skin conditions, many patients experience social stigmatization, shame and social anxiety [3, 10, 11]. A study by Ginsburg and Link [12] revealed that about 20 percent of patients with psoriasis experienced being sent away from sports, hairdressers or swimming facilities because of their skin condition. However, the proportion of patients that suffer from 'the experience of stigmatization' is far greater. Indeed, Lu *et al.* [13] found that about 80 percent of patients with psoriasis and atopic eczema felt stigmatized by others because of their skin disease at least once, 30 percent of which severely. The experience of stigmatization is one of the strongest determinants of perceived restrictions in everyday life [14, 15] and can lead to decreased self-confidence and feelings of shame. These feelings can cause people to isolate themselves and avoid being in public (for example, at restaurants, sports centers or beaches). Additionally, such feelings can lead to fear of interacting with others, which in turn can affect interpersonal relationships [16].

Certain skin conditions that develop at early age, for example atopic eczema, or develop at a certain developmental phase, such as acne, can affect psychosocial development. Children and adolescents who suffer from skin conditions report a lower quality of life compared to peers with other conditions that occur during childhood, such as asthma and diabetes [17]. Apart from complaints of itch and pain this group can also experience emotional and social problems, such as shame, sleep problems, restrictions in hobbies and restrictions in entering into relationships [17, 18]. Additionally, chronic skin conditions do not only affect the child but the whole family, so that parents are found to have lower quality of life and higher rates of psychological distress [19].

A relatively rare category of skin conditions are those in which the complaints are considered mainly psychogenic. Conditions which are characterized by self-harm fall into this category, for example factitious disorder, where patients hurt themselves systematically and repeatedly in order to be diagnosed with a skin condition (this condition is also known as Münchausen's syndrome or dermatitis artefacta) [20, 21]. Furthermore there are several compulsive disorders that express themselves on the skin, such as trichotillomania (the compulsion to pull out one's hair and eyebrows) and skin picking disorder or dermatillomania (the compulsion to continually pick or rub one's skin). Conditions such as delusional infestation, in which patients strongly believe that they are infested by parasites, also fall into this category. Patients suffering from this condition often experience itch and/or pain as well as wounded skin caused by scratching. Despite the psychiatric nature of these conditions, patients suffering from them often visit the dermatologist because of their skin complaints. In recent years more and more attention has been paid to body dysmorphic disorder, in which patients are preoccupied with a supposedly objective deficiency in their appearance, which is often related to their skin. Obsessive preoccupation with one's skin, for example frequently looking at it in the mirror, can also be experienced by patients with for example acne vulgaris or alopecia (excessive hair loss).

PSYCHOSOCIAL FACTORS IN DERMATOLOGICAL CONDITIONS

On average patients with skin conditions have a lower quality of life than the general population. However, there are large differences between individual patients. As in other somatic conditions these differences cannot be explained by the severity of the skin condition alone. Psychosocial factors can influence the onset and/ or the course of certain skin conditions.

About two-thirds of patients with psoriasis and atopic eczema report that stress influences the course of their condition [3, 22, 23]. This influence of stress on the skin is a possible starting point for psychological interventions. For example, improving stress coping mechanisms by means of stress management trainings could affect the severity of a skin condition. The relationship between stress and the course of a condition could in part be explained by the role that the immune system plays in chronic inflammatory skin diseases. More specifically, neuroendocrine and immune mechanisms (for example cortisol and cytokines) can be influenced by stress and can in turn influence chronic skin-related inflammatory activity [22, 24]. Indeed, several prospective studies found a link between stressors and the course of conditions [23 - 25]. Accordingly, in patients with atopic eczema, subjective stress proved to predict disease severity on the following day [26]. Additionally, in patients with psoriasis, high levels of daily stressors were associated with an increase in disease severity and itch four weeks later [24, 25]. Stressors can influence wound healing [27], although this relationship has not been studied in patients with skin conditions. Some correlations have also been found between for example stressors, cortisol and indicators of disease severity [7, 22, 24], however future research is necessary to further investigate these relationships. Stress influences skin conditions, and skin conditions cause stress for the patient resulting in a vicious cycle. Itch is correlated with an increased activity of the autonomic and central nervous system which expresses itself as increased anxiety. Also the visibility of the condition and the perceived stigmatization is a significant stressor for patients. Additionally, many patients report that time-intensive treatments and their impact on everyday life can lead to stressful situations.

An important mediating factor between stressors and disease outcomes is the way patients cope with their condition, including their opinions and attitudes about it, and the perceived support from their environment. Many patients with skin conditions experience feelings of helplessness when trying to cope with their condition. In particular the unpredictable course of a skin condition and the lack of control can make coping more difficult. In line with research on other chronic physical conditions there is some indication that a more passive, avoiding coping style and catastrophizing cognitions can negatively affect the course of a condition and the success of a treatment [7, 8, 25, 28]. Furthermore, studies in people with atopic eczema and psoriasis have revealed connections between perceived helplessness in coping with the condition and decreased physical and psychological well-being [2]. In many physical conditions, perceived social support is an important predictor of long-term functioning. Considering the visibility of skin conditions and their impact on daily life these findings could be especially relevant for skin conditions. However, research on this relationship has so far received relatively little attention [2]. Health behavior can also affect the course of skin conditions. Given that daily skin care with ointments requires a lot of self-reliance, time and effort, following treatment prescriptions is often difficult for dermatological patients. Research shows that approximately 44% of patients do not follow their treatment prescriptions exactly [29, 30]. Besides lack of adherence, lifestyle factors can also affect the course of a chronic physical condition. There are, for example, indications that in patients with chronic ulcer (open wound), healing of venous ulcers can be slowed by lack of exercise and obesity [31].

Increasing attention is paid to scratching behavior as a perpetuating factor of itch in chronic skin conditions [3, 9]. Primarily, scratching is an automatic action to reduce itch. Frequent scratching, however, leads to skin damage and the healing process of these scratching wounds is again accompanied by itch, which may lead to a vicious cycle of itch-scratching problems. Additionally, research in learning theory shows that scratching can lead to a generalized conditioned response to stressors and other environmental stimuli in the long term [9]. In these cases, people scratch not only in response to itch but also as a reaction to stress, anxiety, boredom or other stimuli that have been associated with scratching over time. This scratching behavior can be aggravated by reinforcing factors from the environment. For example, the attention that a child receives from his/her parents can contribute to maintaining the problematic scratching behavior. Through the effects of skin damage due to scratching behavior, this itch-scratch problem can have a significant and persisting influence on the severity of the disease and the effects of dermatological treatments [9, 32].

PSYCHOLOGICAL ASSESSMENT AND DIAGNOSTICS IN DERMATOLOGICAL CONDITIONS

Referral to a psychologist or other psychosocial counselor is common when dermatological interventions have insufficient results, or when there is a possibility of psychosocial problems. In standardized interviews, it is important to identify and assess psychosocial symptoms as well as those factors that can influence the skin condition, such as stressors, health behavior, adherence, social anxiety, itch-scratching problems, or overall coping. Standardized questionnaires can be used in support of the information obtained from the interview in order to determine the right treatment. Several questionnaires with adequate psychometric qualities are available to identify the overall physical, psychological and social well-being of patients with skin conditions. The most widely used questionnaire is the Dermatological Life Quality Index (DLQI) [33], a one-dimensional, dermatology-specific quality of life questionnaire consisting of ten items for which extensive normative data has been published for a wide variety of skin conditions [33]. The more extensive Skindex [34] is a questionnaire which assesses the physical, emotional and social functioning of a patient with the help of several scales, and which is validated for various chronic skin conditions. Additionally, questionnaires for other physical conditions have been adapted to assess chronic skin conditions. For example, the Impact of Chronic Skin Disease on Daily Life (ISDL) [35] which makes it possible to compare how different physical conditions impact psychological and social well-being. A widely used instrument to assess the quality of life in children with skin conditions is the Children's Dermatology Life Quality Index (CDLQI) [36]. In addition to these questionnaires about skin conditions, generic instruments are frequently used such as the Short Form Health Status Survey (SF-36) [37] which can be used to assess the physical and psychological quality of life in people with chronic conditions. A disadvantage of generic questionnaires is that they do not measure specific physical effects of skin conditions, such as itch, and do not make use of available instruments which identify skin-related cognitive and behavioral factors.

Furthermore, instruments are available that measure skin-related cognitive and behavioral factors. The above mentioned ISDL, for example, also measures behavioral factors such as itch-scratching problems, illness cognitions of perceived helplessness and acceptance and the amount of social support. Other similar questionnaires are the Itching Cognitions Questionnaire (ICQ) [38 - 40] which assesses a variety of cognitions about itch such as catastrophizing and the Adjustment to Chronic Skin Diseases Questionnaire (ACS) [41] which measure different skin-related illness cognitions and coping strategies for coping with skin conditions. Additionally, specific questionnaires have been developed to measure the degree of stigmatization [35, 42, 43]. Similar instruments have also been developed for children and adolescents with atopic eczema [44]. Finally, stressors and personality traits are usually measured with generic questionnaires that have been validated for various chronic somatic and mental conditions.

PSYCHOLOGICAL TREATMENTS FOR PATIENTS WITH DERMATOLOGICAL CONDITIONS

Psychological treatments are widely used to improve the psychosocial and physical well-being of people with chronic skin conditions [3, 22]. These interventions vary in the degree to which they attempt to change behaviors. There are unimodal interventions in which single treatments are used, for example psycho-education or relaxation exercises, and multimodal treatments in which a variety of different interventions are applied based on cognitive-behavioral therapy and self-management principles. These interventions usually focus on how patients cope with disease-related factors such as itch, scratching or experienced stigmatization. In this, a distinction can be made between interventions that focus primarily on skin-related psychosocial problems, interventions that focus on itch-scratching problems, and interventions that are focused on psychiatric problems in the dermatological practice. The content of, and scientific evidence for these specific psychological treatments in the different categories will be described below.

Treatments of Skin-Related Psychosocial Problems

Important skin-related factors in chronic skin conditions that can be targeted by psychological treatments are social anxiety, depression, perceived stigmatization and dysfunctional coping strategies, such as avoidance behavior, acceptance and adjustment problems. In these cases, cognitive-behavioral methods are used that have been proven effective for these kinds of problems [3, 22, 45, 46].

Unimodal treatments that consist of psycho-education have so far been used to target psychosocial problems in children and adolescents with skin-conditions and their parents. A review of randomized controlled trials in patients with chronic skin conditions reveals that in particular interventions involving a multidisciplinary team and several meetings, participants reported an improved quality of life and reduced disease severity [47]. One example is the intervention of Staab *et al.* [48] in which a distinction was made between different age groups, and children with atopic eczema and their parents were provided with a structured psycho-education, consisting of six sessions which were led by a multidisciplinary team (among others a dermatologist, a psychologist, a nurse and a dietician). Following this intervention, patients reported reduced disease severity. Similar results were found with educational interventions in adults [47].

Because of the connection between stress-related factors and skin conditions, relaxation exercises and stress-management interventions are frequently used in the treatment of skin conditions. Among the feasible exercises are various relaxation techniques such as progressive relaxation, autogenic training, visualization exercises, biofeedback, but also multimodal interventions which integrate, among others, cognitive restructuring techniques and methods which strengthen problem-solving skills. The rationale behind such interventions is that by changing the stress response one can also influence inflammatory activity and diseases severity. A recent study found that patients with atopic eczema that participated in a short-term stress management training indeed showed a decreased cortisol response during exposure to a psychosocial stressor compared to the control group [49]. However, in this study no effect on the severity of the eczema was found, possibly because the sample was too small or the follow-up too short. There are also indications that patients with psoriasis and atopic eczema benefit from stress-focused relaxation therapy [50], which resulted in decreased disease severity in patients with atopic eczema [51] and a reduction of required phototherapy sessions in patients with psoriasis [52].

Especially in patients with psoriasis and atopic eczema, multimodal cognitive-behavioral treatments have been shown to be effective, for example in improving emotional functioning, reducing disease severity and itching, and increasing the effectiveness of regular dermatological treatments. An example of these treatments is short-term cognitive-behavioral group therapy in patients with psoriasis. In addition to information about the diseases, this short-term group therapy uses stress management, relaxation therapy and cognitive therapy which focuses on disease-related attitudes, social anxiety and perceived stigmatization. In one study patients reported reduced disease severity, less disease-related stress, anxiety and depression compared to the control group directly after the treatment and at a follow-up assessment six month later [53]. Also, a treatment consisting of twelve sessions focusing on education, relaxation, techniques to control scratching, which made use of self-control techniques and habit reversal, stress-management and improvement of communication, was effective in improving the severity of the skin condition [51].

A new development is the application of psychological interventions in the form of education, self-management and cognitive behavioral therapy *via* the Internet (eHealth), which is increasingly used in cognitive-behavioral treatments of patients with chronic somatic conditions, including skin diseases [54, 55]. eHealth has several important advantages, such as a greater reach of care and better access to care, less time consumption and travel costs for the patient and a great flexibility for therapist and patient. There are indications that eHealth interventions can be as effective as face to face treatments for various physical ailments [56]. Additionally, psychological interventions focused on mindfulness and acceptance, which are increasingly used in treating chronic conditions, offer promising possibilities for the psychological treatment of skin conditions [52].

Furthermore, multimodal interventions for children have been developed that make use of education in combination with cognitive behavioral therapy and relaxation therapy [57]. For example, an intervention focused on education, stress management and improvement of social skills in children and adolescents with psoriasis proved effective in improving skin complaints, self-image and social constraints [58]. An example is the Supportive Program for Education, Coping and Training of Parents and Children with Psoriasis and Eczema (SPECTRUM), a multidisciplinary group treatment for children with psoriasis and eczema and their parents. During four meetings led by a dermatologist, a clinical psychologist, and a nurse, it is attempted to increase the self-reliance of children and their parents in dealing with the condition [59].

Treatments of Itch-Scratching Problems

A considerable amount of research has been conducted on the effects of cognitive behavioral treatments specifically focused on itch-scratching problems. In clinical practice, these treatments are frequently applied in combination with psychological treatments for skin-related problems. The primary goal of treatments for itch-scratching problems is to improve the way patients cope with itch and to decrease scratching behavior. In the long-term, it is also expected that itch and the severity of the skin disease is reduced and patients' quality of life improved. The treatments thus have the following two areas of focus: dealing with itch, and dealing with scratching. In dealing with itch, attention has to be paid to the regular application of skin care routines (for example, application of ointments), avoidance of itch-triggering stimuli or situations (for example transpiration, in many skin conditions) and the application of itch- and stress-decreasing measures (for example, relaxation exercises). In dealing with scratching, raising awareness of scratching habits (for example, through registration of scratching behavior) takes a central role and patients are taught different methods to control scratching. The best known method for controlling scratching is 'habit reversal' in which patients learn to replace scratching with an alternative behavior [60]. A basic principle of these treatments is to increase the responsibility and autonomy of the patient in dealing with itch and scratching. For example, through education and registration exercises, patients become aware of early signals of skin deterioration (for example, more itch, scales on the skin, red skin). Subsequently, they try to recognize these signals at an early stage in their daily lives in order to take appropriate action (for example, applying more ointments, protecting the skin by using bandages, adding more relaxation to daily lives), with which further aggravation can be prevented. In case of very severe itch, this intervention can also be combined with pharmacological therapies, such as antihistamines or antidepressants in a very low dosage [61].

Research mainly focuses on multimodal interventions that proved to be effective in reducing disease activity and/ or reducing the degree of itch and scratching in patients with atopic eczema or other chronic skin conditions in adults, children and adolescents [32, 40, 48, 51]. The active mechanisms of these interventions have so far received little attention. It is however known, that in patients with atopic eczema scratch-management methods including habit reversal are effective [62]. Regarding the duration of the treatment, there are indications that in addition to the proven effective treatments that include twelve meetings [51], research suggests that a short-term multidisciplinary group treatment of five meetings can have clinically significant effects in the long-term [32]. The training was provided by a cognitive behavioral therapist and a specialized nurse, using the aforementioned combination of methods aimed at reducing itch-scratching problems [32].

Treatments of Psychiatric Problems in Dermatological Practice

In patients with psychiatric problems and severe psychopathology, such as self-inflicted skin lesions in factitious disorder (dermatitis artefacta), delusional infestation, trichotillomania, skin picking disorder and body dysmorphic disorder, the nature of the condition implies that psychological treatments tend to be more complex and lengthy. In addition to that, the referral to the psychologist or psychiatrist can be a significant challenge, especially in patients with factitious disorder, delusional infestation or body dysmorphic disorder, who can often experience this as a sign of lack of understanding. In these cases, a multidisciplinary psychodermatological approach of the dermatologist and the psychologist/psychiatrist is critical.

For some conditions, it is known that patients benefit from cognitive-behavioral therapy. For example in patients with trichotillomania, behavioral therapies for impulse control, such as habit reversal, have been applied with promising results [63]. Also for skin picking (dermatillomania) effective treatments have been developed, which use among other things habit reversal and cognitive restructuring techniques [64, 65]. For body dysmorphic disorder, effective behavioral therapies have been developed, which focus on exposure to (fear triggering) social stimuli, response prevention (for example looking at oneself in the mirror, omitting superfluous make-up) and changing irrational beliefs and cognitions about one's own appearance [66, 67].

In conditions that have not been researched systematically yet, such as self-inflicted lesions in factitious disorder, cognitive-behavioral approaches are advised in the medical context, aimed at reducing or eliminating self-injurious behavior. In these cases, initial attention has to be paid to building trust between the patient and the dermatologist. The consulting psychologist or psychiatrist is present in the background to carefully assess at which stage of the therapy confrontation is appropriate. It is important that a neutral attitude is adopted towards the self-injurious behavior. In most cases, a psychotherapeutic treatment is focused on, among other things, elucidating the possible functions of this behavior. Learning new coping strategies is necessary to eliminate self-injurious behavior [20]. Especially in delusions such as delusional infestation, these treatments tend to be combined with pharmacotherapy [3, 22].

CONCLUSION

Considering the high prevalence of physical, emotional and social problems in patients with skin conditions, it is crucial that these problems are recognized at an early stage, in order to provide additional psychological care if necessary. However, in the clinical practice of dermatological consultation, limited attention is paid to potential psychosocial consequences of skin conditions and availability of multidisciplinary approaches focusing on systematic screening and corresponding treatments are only incidental [16, 68]. It is therefore of great importance that increased attention is paid to psychological research and clinical applications in the field of dermatology, such as the implementation of screening instruments in dermatological practice. Also, further development, evaluation and implementation of psychological interventions for skin-related problems, itch-scratching problems and psychiatric problems in dermatological practice is important, as the existing evidence shows promising results for physical and psychological functioning in skin patients [46]. Applications through the Internet also offer promising starting points to further facilitate the psychodermatological approach [54 - 56]. In addition, more research is needed to further elucidate the possible interactions between psychological and skin-related (inflammatory-) mechanisms, which will provide possible starting points to further specify psychological and psychopharmocological interventions.

CONFLICT OF INTEREST

An adjusted version of this chapter has previously been published in Dutch as "Spillekom-van Koulil, S. & Evers, A.W.M. (2013). Psychologische behandeling van huidaandoeningen [Psychological treatments of skin diseases]. *Directieve therapie, 33,* 4, 336-361".

ACKNOWLEDGEMENTS

Declared none.

REFERENCES

[1] Verhoeven EW, Kraaimaat FW, van de Kerkhof PC, *et al.* Prevalence of physical symptoms of itch, pain and fatigue in patients with skin diseases in general practice. Br J Dermatol 2007; 156(6): 1346-9. [http://dx.doi.org/10.1111/j.1365-2133.2007.07916.x] [PMID: 17535233]

[2] Evers AW, Lu Y, Duller P, van der Valk PG, Kraaimaat FW, van de Kerkhof PC. Common burden of chronic skin diseases? Contributors to psychological distress in adults with psoriasis and atopic dermatitis. Br J Dermatol 2005; 152(6): 1275-81. [http://dx.doi.org/10.1111/j.1365-2133.2005.06565.x] [PMID: 15948993]

[3] Stangier U, Ehlers A. Stress and anxiety in dermatological disorders. In: Mostofsky DI, Barlow DH, Eds. The management of stress and anxiety in medical disorders. Needham Heights: Allyn & Bacon 2000; pp. 304-43.

[4] Verhoeven EW, Kraaimaat FW, van de Kerkhof PC, *et al.* Psychosocial well-being of patients with skin diseases in general practice. J Eur Acad Dermatol Venereol 2007; 21(5): 662-8. [PMID: 17447981]

[5] Rieder E, Tausk F. Psoriasis, a model of dermatologic psychosomatic disease: psychiatric implications and treatments. Int J Dermatol 2012; 51(1): 12-26. [http://dx.doi.org/10.1111/j.1365-4632.2011.05071.x] [PMID: 22182372]

[6] Dalgard FJ, Gieler U, Tomas-Aragones L, *et al.* The psychological burden of skin diseases: a cross-sectional multicenter study among dermatological out-patients in 13 European countries. J Invest Dermatol 2015; 135(4): 984-91. [http://dx.doi.org/10.1038/jid.2014.530] [PMID: 25521458]

[7] Fortune DG, Richards HL, Griffiths CE. Psychologic factors in psoriasis: consequences, mechanisms, and interventions. Dermatol Clin 2005; 23(4): 681-94.
[http://dx.doi.org/10.1016/j.det.2005.05.022] [PMID: 16112445]

[8] Fortune DG, Richards HL, Kirby B, *et al.* Psychological distress impairs clearance of psoriasis in patients treated with photochemotherapy. Arch Dermatol 2003; 139(6): 752-6.
[http://dx.doi.org/10.1001/archderm.139.6.752] [PMID: 12810506]

[9] Yosipovitch G, Greaves MW, McGlone F, Eds. Itch. New York: Marcel Dekker 2003.

[10] Ginsburg IH, Link BG. Feelings of stigmatization in patients with psoriasis. J Am Acad Dermatol 1989; 20(1): 53-63.
[http://dx.doi.org/10.1016/S0190-9622(89)70007-4] [PMID: 2913081]

[11] Schmid-Ott G, Künsebeck HW, Jäger B, *et al.* Significance of the stigmatization experience of psoriasis patients: a 1-year follow-up of the illness and its psychosocial consequences in men and women. Acta Derm Venereol 2005; 85(1): 27-32.
[http://dx.doi.org/10.1080/00015550410021583] [PMID: 15848987]

[12] Ginsburg IH, Link BG. Psychosocial consequences of rejection and stigma feelings in psoriasis patients. Int J Dermatol 1993; 32(8): 587-91.
[http://dx.doi.org/10.1111/j.1365-4362.1993.tb05031.x] [PMID: 8407075]

[13] Lu Y, Duller P, Van Der Valk PG, *et al.* Helplessness as predictor of perceived stigmatization in patients with psoriasis and atopic dermatitis. Dermatol Psychosom 2003; 4(3): 146-50.
[http://dx.doi.org/10.1159/000073991]

[14] Richards HL, Fortune DG, Griffiths CE, Main CJ. The contribution of perceptions of stigmatisation to disability in patients with psoriasis. J Psychosom Res 2001; 50(1): 11-5.
[http://dx.doi.org/10.1016/S0022-3999(00)00210-5] [PMID: 11259795]

[15] Vardy D, Besser A, Amir M, Gesthalter B, Biton A, Buskila D. Experiences of stigmatization play a role in mediating the impact of disease severity on quality of life in psoriasis patients. Br J Dermatol 2002; 147(4): 736-42.
[http://dx.doi.org/10.1046/j.1365-2133.2002.04899.x] [PMID: 12366421]

[16] Sampogna F, Picardi A, Melchi CF, Pasquini P, Abeni D. The impact of skin diseases on patients: comparing dermatologists' opinions with research data collected on their patients. Br J Dermatol 2003; 148(5): 989-95.
[http://dx.doi.org/10.1046/j.1365-2133.2003.05306.x] [PMID: 12786831]

[17] Beattie PE, Lewis-Jones MS. A comparative study of impairment of quality of life in children with skin disease and children with other chronic childhood diseases. Br J Dermatol 2006; 155(1): 145-51.
[http://dx.doi.org/10.1111/j.1365-2133.2006.07185.x] [PMID: 16792766]

[18] de Jager ME, De Jong EM, Evers AW, Van De Kerkhof PC, Seyger MM. The burden of childhood psoriasis. Pediatr Dermatol 2011; 28(6): 736-7.
[http://dx.doi.org/10.1111/j.1525-1470.2011.01489.x] [PMID: 21692835]

[19] Warschburger P, Buchholz HT, Petermann F. Psychological adjustment in parents of young children with atopic dermatitis: which factors predict parental quality of life? Br J Dermatol 2004; 150(2): 304-11.

[http://dx.doi.org/10.1111/j.1365-2133.2004.05743.x] [PMID: 14996102]

[20] Koblenzer CS, Gupta R. Neurotic excoriations and dermatitis artefacta. Semin Cutan Med Surg 2013; 32(2): 95-100.
[http://dx.doi.org/10.12788/j.sder.0008] [PMID: 24049967]

[21] Gieler U, Consoli SG, Tomás-Aragones L, *et al.* Self-inflicted lesions in dermatology: terminology and classification--a position paper from the European Society for Dermatology and Psychiatry (ESDaP). Acta Derm Venereol 2013; 93(1): 4-12.
[PMID: 23303467]

[22] Koo JY, Lee CS, Eds. Psychocutaneous Medicine. New York: Marcel Dekker 2003.

[23] Picardi A, Abeni D. Stressful life events and skin diseases: disentangling evidence from myth. Psychother Psychosom 2001; 70(3): 118-36.
[http://dx.doi.org/10.1159/000056237] [PMID: 11340413]

[24] Evers AW, Verhoeven EW, Kraaimaat FW, *et al.* How stress gets under the skin: cortisol and stress reactivity in psoriasis. Br J Dermatol 2010; 163(5): 986-91.
[http://dx.doi.org/10.1111/j.1365-2133.2010.09984.x] [PMID: 20716227]

[25] Verhoeven EW, Kraaimaat FW, Jong EM, Schalkwijk J, van de Kerkhof PC, Evers AW. Effect of daily stressors on psoriasis: a prospective study. J Invest Dermatol 2009; 129(8): 2075-7.
[http://dx.doi.org/10.1038/jid.2008.460] [PMID: 19194471]

[26] King RM, Wilson GV. Use of a diary technique to investigate psychosomatic relations in atopic dermatitis. J Psychosom Res 1991; 35(6): 697-706.
[http://dx.doi.org/10.1016/0022-3999(91)90120-D] [PMID: 1791583]

[27] Christian LM, Graham JE, Padgett DA, *et al.* Stress and Wound Healing Neuroimmunomodulat 2006; 13(5-6): 337-46.

[28] Scharloo M, Kaptein AA, Weinman J, Bergman W, Vermeer BJ, Rooijmans HG. Patients' illness perceptions and coping as predictors of functional status in psoriasis: a 1-year follow-up. Br J Dermatol 2000; 142(5): 899-907.
[http://dx.doi.org/10.1046/j.1365-2133.2000.03469.x] [PMID: 10809846]

[29] Renzi C, Picardi A, Abeni D, *et al.* Association of dissatisfaction with care and psychiatric morbidity with poor treatment compliance. Arch Dermatol 2002; 138(3): 337-42.
[http://dx.doi.org/10.1001/archderm.138.3.337] [PMID: 11902984]

[30] Serup J, Lindblad AK, Maroti M, *et al.* To follow or not to follow dermatological treatment--a review of the literature. Acta Derm Venereol 2006; 86(3): 193-7.
[http://dx.doi.org/10.2340/00015555-0073] [PMID: 16710573]

[31] Heinen MM, van Achterberg T, op Reimer WS, van de Kerkhof PC, de Laat E. Venous leg ulcer patients: a review of the literature on lifestyle and pain-related interventions. J Clin Nurs 2004; 13(3): 355-66.
[http://dx.doi.org/10.1046/j.1365-2702.2003.00887.x] [PMID: 15009338]

[32] Evers AW, Duller P, de Jong EM, *et al.* Effectiveness of a multidisciplinary itch-coping training programme in adults with atopic dermatitis. Acta Derm Venereol 2009; 89(1): 57-63.
[http://dx.doi.org/10.2340/00015555-0556] [PMID: 19197543]

[33] Lewis V, Finlay AY. 10 years experience of the dermatology life quality index (DLQI). J Investig Dermatol Symp Proc 2004; 9(2): 169-80. [http://dx.doi.org/10.1111/j.1087-0024.2004.09113.x] [PMID: 15083785]

[34] Chren M-M, Lasek RJ, Quinn LM, Mostow EN, Zyzanski SJ. Skindex, a quality-of-life measure for patients with skin disease: reliability, validity, and responsiveness. J Invest Dermatol 1996; 107(5): 707-13. [http://dx.doi.org/10.1111/1523-1747.ep12365600] [PMID: 8875954]

[35] Evers AW, Duller P, van de Kerkhof PC, *et al.* The impact of chronic skin disease on daily life (ISDL): A generic and dermatology specific health instrument. Br J Dermatol 2008; 158(1): 101-8. [PMID: 17999699]

[36] Lewis-Jones MS, Finlay AY. The Children's Dermatology Life Quality Index (CDLQI): initial validation and practical use. Br J Dermatol 1995; 132(6): 942-9. [http://dx.doi.org/10.1111/j.1365-2133.1995.tb16953.x] [PMID: 7662573]

[37] Ware JE Jr, Sherbourne CD. The MOS 36-item short-form health survey (SF-36). I. Conceptual framework and item selection. Med Care 1992; 30(6): 473-83. [http://dx.doi.org/10.1097/00005650-199206000-00002] [PMID: 1593914]

[38] Ehlers A, Stangier U, Dohn D, *et al.* Kognitive faktoren beim juckreiz: Entwicklung und zalidierung eines fragebogens. Verhaltenstherapie 1993; 3(2): 112-9. [http://dx.doi.org/10.1159/000258752]

[39] Huizinga J, van Os-Medendorp H, Ros WJ, Grypdonck M, Lablans JA, Dijkstra GJ. Validation of the Dutch version of the itching cognitions questionnaire. J Nurs Meas 2012; 20(1): 35-46. [http://dx.doi.org/10.1891/1061-3749.20.1.35] [PMID: 22679708]

[40] van Os-Medendorp H, Eland-de Kok PC, Ros WJ, Bruijnzeel-Koomen CA, Grypdonck M. The nursing programme 'Coping with itch': a promising intervention for patients with chronic pruritic skin diseases. J Clin Nurs 2007; 16(7): 1238-46. [http://dx.doi.org/10.1111/j.1365-2702.2007.01590.x] [PMID: 17584341]

[41] Stangier U, Ehlers A, Gieler U. Measuring adjustment to chronic skin disorders: validation of a self-report measure. Psychol Assess 2003; 15(4): 532-49. [http://dx.doi.org/10.1037/1040-3590.15.4.532] [PMID: 14692848]

[42] Lawrence JW, Fauerbach JA, Heinberg LJ, Doctor M, Thombs BD. The reliability and validity of the Perceived Stigmatization Questionnaire (PSQ) and the Social Comfort Questionnaire (SCQ) among an adult burn survivor sample. Psychol Assess 2006; 18(1): 106-11. [http://dx.doi.org/10.1037/1040-3590.18.1.106] [PMID: 16594819]

[43] Schmid-Ott G, Jaeger B, Kuensebeck HW, Ott R, Lamprecht F. Dimensions of stigmatization in patients with psoriasis in a "Questionnaire on Experience with Skin Complaints'. Dermatology (Basel) 1996; 193(4): 304-10. [http://dx.doi.org/10.1159/000246275] [PMID: 8993954]

[44] Kupfer J, Keins P, Brosig B, *et al.* Development of questionnaires on coping with disease and itching cognitions for children and adolescents with atopic eczema. Dermatol Psychosom 2003; 4(2): 79-85. [http://dx.doi.org/10.1159/000072196]

[45] Chida Y, Steptoe A, Hirakawa N, Sudo N, Kubo C. The effects of psychological intervention on atopic dermatitis. A systematic review and meta-analysis. Int Arch Allergy Immunol 2007; 144(1): 1-9. [http://dx.doi.org/10.1159/000101940] [PMID: 17449959]

[46] Lavda AC, Webb TL, Thompson AR. A meta-analysis of the effectiveness of psychological interventions for adults with skin conditions. Br J Dermatol 2012; 167(5): 970-9. [http://dx.doi.org/10.1111/j.1365-2133.2012.11183.x] [PMID: 22924999]

[47] de Bes J, Legierse CM, Prinsen CA, de Korte J. Patient education in chronic skin diseases: a systematic review. Acta Derm Venereol 2011; 91(1): 12-7. [http://dx.doi.org/10.2340/00015555-1022] [PMID: 21264451]

[48] Staab D, Diepgen TL, Fartasch M, *et al.* Age related, structured educational programmes for the management of atopic dermatitis in children and adolescents: multicentre, randomised controlled trial. BMJ 2006; 332(7547): 933-8. [http://dx.doi.org/10.1136/bmj.332.7547.933] [PMID: 16627509]

[49] Schut C, Weik U, Tews N, Gieler U, Deinzer R, Kupfer J. Psychophysiological effects of stress management in patients with atopic dermatitis: a randomized controlled trial. Acta Derm Venereol 2013; 93(1): 57-61. [PMID: 22983681]

[50] Fordham B, Griffiths CE, Bundy C. Can stress reduction interventions improve psoriasis? A review. Psychol Health Med 2013; 18(5): 501-14. [http://dx.doi.org/10.1080/13548506.2012.736625] [PMID: 23116223]

[51] Ehlers A, Stangier U, Gieler U. Treatment of atopic dermatitis: a comparison of psychological and dermatological approaches to relapse prevention. J Consult Clin Psychol 1995; 63(4): 624-35. [http://dx.doi.org/10.1037/0022-006X.63.4.624] [PMID: 7673540]

[52] Kabat-Zinn J, Wheeler E, Light T, *et al.* Influence of a mindfulness meditation-based stress reduction intervention on rates of skin clearing in patients with moderate to severe psoriasis undergoing phototherapy (UVB) and photochemotherapy (PUVA). Psychosom Med 1998; 60(5): 625-32. [http://dx.doi.org/10.1097/00006842-199809000-00020] [PMID: 9773769]

[53] Fortune DG, Richards HL, Kirby B, Bowcock S, Main CJ, Griffiths CE. A cognitive-behavioural symptom management programme as an adjunct in psoriasis therapy. Br J Dermatol 2002; 146(3): 458-65. [http://dx.doi.org/10.1046/j.1365-2133.2002.04622.x] [PMID: 11952546]

[54] van Cranenburgh OD, Smets EM, de Rie MA, Sprangers MA, de Korte J. A Web-based, educational, quality-of-life intervention for patients with a chronic skin disease: feasibility and acceptance in routine dermatological practice. Acta Derm Venereol 2015; 95(1): 51-6. [http://dx.doi.org/10.2340/00015555-1872] [PMID: 24733369]

[55] Bundy C, Pinder B, Bucci S, Reeves D, Griffiths CE, Tarrier N. A novel, web-based, psychological intervention for people with psoriasis: the electronic Targeted Intervention for Psoriasis (eTIPs) study. Br J Dermatol 2013; 169(2): 329-36. [http://dx.doi.org/10.1111/bjd.12350] [PMID: 23551271]

[56] van Beugen S, Ferwerda M, Hoeve D, *et al.* A meta-analytic review of internet-based cognitive

behavioral therapy for patients with chronic somatic conditions. J Med Internet Res 2014; 16(3): e88. [http://dx.doi.org/10.2196/jmir.2777] [PMID: 24675372]

[57] Ersser SJ, Cowdell F, Latter S, *et al.* Psychological and educational interventions for atopic eczema in children. Cochrane Database Syst Rev 2014; 1: CD004054. [PMID: 24399641]

[58] Scheewe S, Schmidt S, Petermann F, *et al.* Long-term efficacy of an inpatient rehabilitation with integrated patient education program for children and adolescents with psoriasis. Dermatol Psychosom 2001; 2(1): 16-21. [http://dx.doi.org/10.1159/000049632]

[59] Oostveen AM, Spillekom-van Koulil S, Otero ME, Klompmaker W, Evers AW, Seyger MM. Development and design of a multidisciplinary training program for outpatient children and adolescents with psoriasis and their parents. J Dermatolog Treat 2013; 24(1): 60-3. [http://dx.doi.org/10.3109/09546634.2012.672707] [PMID: 22390570]

[60] Grillo M, Long R, Long D. Habit reversal training for the itch-scratch cycle associated with pruritic skin conditions. *Dermatology nursing/Dermatology Nurses'*. Association 2007; 19(3): 243-8.

[61] Tey HL, Wallengren J, Yosipovitch G. Psychosomatic factors in pruritus. Clin Dermatol 2013; 31(1): 31-40. [http://dx.doi.org/10.1016/j.clindermatol.2011.11.004] [PMID: 23245971]

[62] Melin L, Frederiksen T, Noren P, Swebilius BG. Behavioural treatment of scratching in patients with atopic dermatitis. Br J Dermatol 1986; 115(4): 467-74. [http://dx.doi.org/10.1111/j.1365-2133.1986.tb06241.x] [PMID: 3778815]

[63] van Minnen A, Hoogduin KA, Keijsers GP, Hellenbrand I, Hendriks GJ. Treatment of trichotillomania with behavioral therapy or fluoxetine: a randomized, waiting-list controlled study. Arch Gen Psychiatry 2003; 60(5): 517-22. [http://dx.doi.org/10.1001/archpsyc.60.5.517] [PMID: 12742873]

[64] Schuck K, Keijsers GP, Rinck M. The effects of brief cognitive-behaviour therapy for pathological skin picking: A randomized comparison to wait-list control. Behav Res Ther 2011; 49(1): 11-7. [http://dx.doi.org/10.1016/j.brat.2010.09.005] [PMID: 20934685]

[65] Teng EJ, Woods DW, Twohig MP. Habit reversal as a treatment for chronic skin picking: a pilot investigation. Behav Modif 2006; 30(4): 411-22. [http://dx.doi.org/10.1177/0145445504265707] [PMID: 16723422]

[66] Prazeres AM, Nascimento AL, Fontenelle LF. Cognitive-behavioral therapy for body dysmorphic disorder: a review of its efficacy. Neuropsychiatr Dis Treat 2013; 9: 307-16. [PMID: 23467711]

[67] Ipser JC, Sander C, Stein DJ. Pharmacotherapy and psychotherapy for body dysmorphic disorder. Cochrane Database Syst Rev 2009; 1(1): CD005332. [PMID: 19160252]

[68] Luteijn MC, Boonstra HE, Castelen G, *et al.* Psychodermatologie in de Nederlandse dermatologische praktijk. Nederland Tijdschr Dermatol Venereol 2011; 21: 545-9.

CHAPTER 9

Psychoanalysis in Psychodermatological Diseases

Jorge C. Ulnik*

Universidad de Buenos Aires. Facultad de Psicología. Cátedra Fisiopatología y Enfermedades Psicosomáticas Buenos Aires, Argentina. Asociación Psicoanalítica Argentina. Universidad de Buenos Aires. Facultad de Medicina. Departamento de Psiquiatría y Salud Mental. Buenos Aires, Argentina

Abstract: From a psychoanalytical point of view, almost all dermatological disorders can be considered psychodermatological disorders, because psychoanalytical conception of psychosomatics is not based on the absence of an organic aetiology, or on the real somatic condition of the disease. In all of them – either self inflicted or not, delusional or real, chronic or acute - a psychodynamic approach can be made and can turn out useful, depending more on the patient than on the disorder itself.

Psychoanalytic evaluation can contribute to the dermatologic practice at many different levels: a) establishing the level of psychological/psychiatric functioning during the consultation; b) typifying the kind of unconscious conflicts and emotions that the patient expresses through his/her complaints and symptoms; c) detecting the defence mechanisms that the patient uses to cope with reality, with stress and with his disease; d) choosing the treatment taking into account the unconscious preferences and meanings of the prescriptions; and e) giving skills to improve doctor-patient relationship.

What the psychoanalyst hears in the doctor's consulting room gives him the possibility to infer that there are unconscious factors which play a role in the motive and time of consultation, the self-destructive patterns of behaviour that worsen the disease, the kind of complaint or suffering privileged by the patient, the acceptance or rejection of a treatment or a medicine and even the location of the lesions.

Keywords: Allergy, Attachment, Doctor-patient relationship, Ego-skin, Emotional expression, Medical psychology, Psoriasis, Psychoanalysis, Psychodermatology, Psychodynamic psychotherapy, Psychosomatics,

* **Corresponding author Jorge C. Ulnik:** Malabia 2255, 2°B, (C1425) Ciudad de Buenos Aires, Argentina; Phone: + 54 11 4 832 5798, Fax: + 54 11 4832 5798; E-mail: jorgeulnik@gmail.com.

Klas Nordlind & Anna Zalewska-Janowska (Eds.)

Psychosomatic diseases, Self-injuring, Skin.

INTRODUCTION

The Skin Patients In Session: Some Transference-Counter Transference Events

A dermatologist referred Magdalena to a psychoanalyst because she was not improving of a chronic eczema, with location in various parts of the body but mainly on her face.

At the beginning of the treatment, her speech was centered on physical complaints, mostly itching and edema. She blushed at some interpretations offered by her psychoanalyst. Many times she stands up to fetch moisturiser, ready to use in a small bottle, and puts it on her face to soothe her itching. Once she has done this, she lies back on the couch and continues talking as if there had been no interruption whatsoever.

Peter, a psoriasis patient, always leaves silver scales of epidermis which stand out against the black leather of the couch. Could we term these phenomena "Skin in psychoanalysis" [1]?

The psychoanalyst would probably reply "no". Peter's psoriasis is genetically determined; his skin comes off in small pieces and there is nothing he can do about it. Magdalena, on the other hand, is allergic and itching is the consequence of her skin disease.

However, the psychoanalyst is feeling upset: he must clean the couch before the next patient arrives; he even considers the possibility of getting a cover for it to be used whenever Peter comes to therapy. While he washes his hands he feels he can hardly keep himself from telling Magdalena not to touch her face during the session. He is feeling upset and anxious: he cannot think "in depth". He might even feel itchy!

Might not his feelings be attributed to counter-transference? Do somatic conditions pose a limit to psychoanalysis?

Peter has an appointment with the dermatologist after his session. While he undresses for the physical exam he leaves a pile of scales on the floor. The dermatologist asks him how he is doing and Peter, pointing to the scales on the floor, replies, “look, there I am”.

What Peter sees in his own scales is himself, as if he was another who leaves traces everywhere. This other “presence” is disavowed by his dermatologist and his psychoanalyst, who just hoover the floor, as Peter’s wife always does, and put Peter’s “other me”, which, incidentally, is torn to pieces, in the rubbish bin.

I learned this from a patient with psoriasis who spoke of her divorced mother saying “If I moved in with Dad, Mum would fall to bits”, while her skin came off in small pieces.

Another one, usually splits herself: One self is the woman: a woman who wears women’s clothes, goes to the hairdresser, and dedicates time to her makeup. The other self is the psoriasis patient: the one who wears “unisex” clothes of light colours, never goes to the hairdresser, and wastes a lot of time moisturizing herself and hiding her body.

“Medical scientific papers claim that one third of the population who consults with a dermatologist suffers from psychological problems and yet, at the same time they claim that cognitive-behavioural therapy is the treatment of choice. Is it that psychoanalysis has no say within this field? Indeed, there are several multidisciplinary societies of psychiatry and dermatology in the United States and in Europe where the voice of psychoanalysis can barely be heard. However, in our present cultural context, where interdisciplinary work is essential and where a piercing or a tattoo grant a feeling of identity to youths whose subjectivity is at risk, the issue of the skin seems to be receiving a lot of attention and we psychoanalysts must bear in mind that Freud used to consider it “the erogenous zone par excellence”, and that it was also the entrance and the exit door for many emotions and situations which mark us” [1].

WHAT IS PSYCHOANALYSIS?

Since there are many current psychoanalytic schools of thought and different theoretical orientations, we will define the psychoanalysis taking and quoting a few extracts from the website of the International Psychoanalytical Association (IPA).

"Psychoanalysis is a treatment approach based on the observation that individuals are often unaware of many of the factors that determine their emotions and behaviour. These unconscious factors may be the source of considerable distress and unhappiness, sometimes in the form of recognizable symptoms and at other times as troubling personality traits, difficulties in work and/or in love relationships, or disturbances in mood and self-esteem.

As these forces are unconscious, the advice of friends and family, the reading of self-help books, or even the most determined efforts of will, often fail to provide relief" [2].

"Psychoanalytic treatment can reveal how these unconscious factors affect current relationships and patterns of behaviour, trace them back to their historical origins, show how they have changed and developed over time, and help the individual to deal better with the realities of adult life.

In the course of intensive psychoanalytic treatment, the "internal world" of the analysand becomes available for experience and exploration by the analysand and analyst together" [2].

"Psychoanalysis, by its very nature, delves into the world of the unconscious mind. It operates on the basis that our early experiences – of whatever nature – strongly influence how our minds develop and how we interact with the other people around us" [2].

"Analysis is a partnership between patient and analyst, in the course of which the patient becomes aware of the underlying sources of his or her difficulties not simply intellectually, but emotionally - by re-experiencing them with the analyst. As the patient speaks, hints of the unconscious sources of current difficulties gradually begin to appear - in certain repetitive patterns of behaviour, in the subjects which the patient finds hard to talk about, in the ways the patient relates to the analyst" [2].

Psychoanalytic Psychotherapy, involves in general (but not necessarily) less sessions per week than orthodox psychoanalysis. Some patients start with one session a week, and not necessarily lie on the couch. This is the kind of psychoanalytic approach more frequently applied with skin patients referred by dermatologists.

Children psychoanalysis is very important as a model, because it works not only through words, but also through drawings and fantasy play. This technique was the starting point for the use or art therapy and drawings analysis that could be used with in a psychosomatic approach.

So far, we've talked about what psychoanalysis is. But ... can psychoanalysis be used in the treatment of patients with skin disorders who go to the dermatologist´s office?

WHAT ABOUT PSYCHOANALYSIS AND DERMATOLOGY?

The allusions to the skin within psychoanalytic theory are manifold, and the authors who have written about this subject within post-Freudian psychoanalysis are several as well. In addition, the skin is usually an “entrance door” for all those of who become involved in the psychosomatic problem and, when it is time to offer clinical examples, eczema [3, 4], psoriasis [5], hives, urticaria [6] and other dermatoses are usually included.

We will divide the answer for the question above in five issues: 1) Theory 2) Referral 3) Dimensions of the diagnosis 4) Skin Symptoms and pathologies and 5) Therapy

1. Theory

There are many psychoanalytic statements that link the psyche and the skin, either directly or indirectly.

Freud discovered that the unconscious mind has a strong influence – an auto-plastic one – on the body and its functioning, and he also stated that “ ...the Ego is first and foremost a bodily ego; it is not merely a surface entity, but it is itself the projection of a surface” [7].

Conceptualizing the Ego as a bodily ego and as a projection of a surface immediately links the Ego with the skin and shows us how similar the skin functions and the Ego ones are.

Limit; container; support; barrier of protection anti-stimuli; screen that displays to the external the state of the inner world; integration of different sensations in a whole (inter-sensoriality); representative of own identity through the Inscription of tactile sensorial traces and by incisions, scarring, paintings, tattoos, makeup, hair styles.

According to D Anzieu, the psyche develops taking as its starting point a basis provided by corporal experiences of a biological nature in which the skin plays a fundamental role. He also says that "The more altered the Ego of the patient is, the deeper and more serious the skin disease he might suffer could be" [8].

In Studies on Hysteria, Freud explored a fantastic anatomy adding to the body representation in medicine, a biographic focus in which language, dreams, sexuality, unconscious wishes and the relationship with the doctor play a fundamental role. In spite of being invisible to the gaze, this anatomy has its fundamental piece on the skin. A piece that has the status – given by Freud – of "erotogenic zone par excellence" [9].

In the psychoanalytical conception, body parts, organs, actions and functioning are engaged with primitive feelings and archaic fantasies [10]. It´s psychosomatic approach links the skin and the unconscious psyche in many different ways, as can be seen in the following quotes: "When we touch a spot, we awake a memory that can evoke a series of historical events and repressed ideas" [11]. "He that has eyes to see and ears to hear may convince himself that no mortal can keep a secret. If his lips are silent, he chatters with his finger-tips; betrayal oozes out of him at every pore. And thus the task of making conscious the most hidden recesses of the mind is one which it is quite possible to accomplish" [12].

After Freud, other psychoanalysts not only in the past but actually have talked about psychological problems that are related to the functions of the skin or have mentioned functions, pathologies and psychological defences that can be compared with or even expressed through alterations in the form and function of the skin. For example, according to E. Bick, "In its most primitive form the parts of the personality are felt to have no binding force amongst themselves and must therefore be held together in a way that is experienced by them passively, by the skin functioning as a boundary" [13].

But this internal function – that of containing the parts of the Self – initially depends on the relationship with another person who must be experienced as capable of fulfilling that function. On the contrary, confusions regarding identity shall take place, and a seudo independence shall be developed, using the hyper activity or muscular development as a "second skin": a substitute for the failed skin container function [13].

Psychoanalysis stresses the importance of the early gazing relationship and of the skin-to-skin contact between mother and baby. A Lemma – talking about body modification – described an axis constituted by touch and vision that underpinnes the earliest physical experiences. She says that "Where there are difficulties in the earliest gaze-touch relationship with the object of desire, it can prove impossible to feel at home in one's own body" [14] and this "...represents an important area of developmental deficit that creates particular vulnerabilities in the integration of the body self into the person´s sense of who they are"[14]. Thus, identity problems occur and body modification could be sought by people to solve these problems with such procedures.

According to Lemma there are three phantasies underpinning the pursuit of body modification: a) The reclaiming phantasy: The body modification serves the function of rescuing the self from an alien presence felt to now reside within the body. This phantasy therefore concerns the *expulsion* from the body of an object felt to be alien or polluting. b) The self-made phantasy: expresses an envious attack on the object. The self believes that it can create itself, thereby circumventing the object, and hence any experience of dependency, and c) The perfect match phantasy: create a perfect, ideal body that will guarantee the other's love and desire.

Beyond Lemma´s statements, we think that skin modifications by self inflicted lesions or even by real skin diseases also satisfy these phantasies.

S. Consoli [15] has stressed the importance of tenderness in the psychic development and in the physical treatment and the psychotherapy of skin patients. She enriched concepts like stress and quality of life analysing them with psychoanalytic contributions: overdetermination of symptoms, atemporal functioning in stress trigger factors, transference and counter transference in doctor-patient relationship, *etc.*

C. Koblenzer 1986, 1995 has published numerous case reports obtaining remissions through insight psychotherapy on patients with recalcitrant dermophaties who didn't have success with traditional dermatologic treatments. She mentions cases in which improvement happened after verbalization and awareness of feelings of guilt, rage and abandonment [16, 17].

F. Poot has described family interactions that have an important role in the psychodynamics of skin patients [18].

D. Pines describes and discusses the psychic predicament of female patients who have suffered from infantile eczema during the first year of life. After drawing on direct observations from her previous experience as a consultant dermatologist in a women's hospital she analyses a patient with a history of this disease. Focusing on transference-countertransference problems she finds a basic disturbance in the earliest mother–infant relationship [19].

2. Referral

What is the reality faced by the dermatologist in his/her daily clinical practice?

1) Psychological variables and stressful life events can trigger or worsen cutaneous symptoms and skin diseases. 2) Emotional implications, psychosocial consequences and anxious-depressive syndromes, can occur secondary to many skin disorders. 3) Patients with primarily psychiatric disorders can visit a dermatologist as their first medical consultation.4) Patients are frequently dissatisfied with traditional medical therapies. They actively seek alternative approaches either to complement or substitute standard treatments. 5) "Most dermatologists have neither the training nor the time for nonpharmacologic treatments" [20].

Facing this reality, the dermatologist tries to refer the patient to a psychiatrist, psychologist or psychoanalyst depending on the severity of the problem and his/her preferences. But the result is disappointing, because usually skin patients refuse the "psy" referral.

Why does it happen?

Difficulties in the Referral to Psychotherapy Treatment

Socio-Cultural Factors

Our culture, focused as it is on the present, proposes magical and immediate solutions to problems and brings the work of introspection to disrepute.

The Degree of Awareness of Psychological Suffering and Feelings

There are patients suffering from chronic dermopathies who have little, if any, awareness of psychological suffering. They are therefore unwilling to commit themselves to treatment, unless they are promised to be healed magically. Some patients fear not being considered a "real" patient or a trustful person. –*"If doctors refer me to a shrink, it means they don't believe me"*. In the same way, others fear being considered crazy or psychiatric patients, and therefore rejected by society. For some people, emotional illness is more of a stigma than a skin disease. They don´t want to take psychiatric medication. Skin disorders are close to stigmatization feeling and psychiatric disorders too. So, changing the stigma is not a solution for the patient's point of view.

Moreover, if a patient has the assumption that healthy adults should be able to work things out on their own, seeking psycho therapeutic help appears to him/her as a sign of weakness more than the disease does. These patients have the tendency to be out of touch with their feelings.

The Kinds of Relationship they Establish

Certain patients, whom we will term "evacuative", usually establish a too confident relationship either with the staff (such as the secretary or the nurse) or the doctor as a means of catharsis. In this way they remove their feelings of anxiety or depression.

Other patients, whom I shall call "dwellers" [21] settle themselves in the waiting room long before the time of their appointment and just linger over, reading the paper, eating, using the toilet or working as if they were in the living-room of their own house.

Infantile, dependent and demanding patients wish the physician took over in a parental fashion and relieved them of the burden [22].

These kinds of patients are usually reluctant to accept the referral to psychotherapy because they obtain, in a parasitical way, benefits from the institutions they attend and from the staff working there.

The Psycho-Somatic Dissociation

Many times, painful emotions and weaknesses are hidden and at the same time expressed by the skin disease. In these cases the fear is that these hidden feelings arise to be experienced. "The feelings you buried were painful or else you'd never have buried them. It's like trying to solve a mystery while you secretly fear that the criminal will prove to be yourself" [23].

In some cases, there are more structural problems, and the aim to maintain the psycho – somatic dissociation, is necessary for the avoidance of a confusional (disturbing) feeling and the support of an apparent mental coherence.

Practical Factors

Usually people go to a therapist's office for psychotherapy sessions. But the skin patient goes to the psychotherapist with the same aim that he or she goes to the doctor: get rid of the skin disorder. So, when the psycho therapist suggests that psychotherapy sessions are needed and the result is not warranted, the patient is disappointed.

Patients usually voice objections such as:

- They anticipate that in general psychological and psychoanalytical treatments will be long.

- They are not told in advance when therapy will be over.
- The high frequency of sessions (even if they are once a week).
- The fact that health insurance plans do not cover psychoanalytic treatments.
- The cost of psychological interviews, which must be added to the general cost of treatment.

Almost all of these difficulties described above could appear with any psychotherapy or psychiatric intervention and are not exclusively a problem with psychoanalysis. But some of them can only be worked by a trained psychoanalyst with experience in psychodermatology and/or psychosomatics since the scope of psychoanalysis includes as one of its main issues the analysis of resistances and the transference[1].

A dermatologist may wonder: When is it recommendable the referral to a psychoanalyst?

The referral is recommendable when the patient expresses actual conflicts such us with family, doctor, at work, *etc.* either related or not with the skin disease; when he or she has "psy" motivation (very important!); when the doctor identifies psychosocial trigger factors in the onset and /or the evolution of the skin disease; when a low quality of life is detected and finally, when there are difficulties in treatment: acceptance of the doctor´s prescriptions, poor response to medication, bad compliance, *etc.*

Psychoanalysis functions better in neurotic organizations of the personality, but sometimes psychotic organizations could improve or at least get a stabilization.

Comorbidities, urgency, and little time available suggest other options.

3. Dimensions of Diagnosis

What or who will be treated with psychotherapy?

When we say: "Dermatitis Artefacta is treated with ...."; "Effects of psychologic interventions on ...psoriasis" or "Setting a service for adult epidermolysis bullosa [24] we are thinking that <u>a dermatologic disease</u> is what must be treated

If we focus on anxiety, depression and psychiatric symptoms, they can be treated independently of the dermatologic disease. Although the causes are different, depression is depression either in psoriasis or in alopecia areata.

Therefore, when making a decision about the referral to the psychologist, the psychoanalyst or the psychiatrist, both clinical (disease-specific) indications and general (psychotherapy-specific) indications should be taken into consideration, case by case with a diagnosis of the underlying psychiatric functioning. (Neurotic, borderline, Psychotic) [25].

Levels of Diagnosis

An understanding of the nature and expected course of the dermatosis is of great value to the psychoanalyst. Thus, he/she should know, the somatic disease diagnosis preferably from the patient´s dermatologist.

At the same time, obtaining the psychiatric diagnosis is also fundamental. (Example: if the patient is depressed: is he/she suffering a bipolar disorder? dysthymia? adaptative disorder? Are organic factors playing a role? Is he/she taking medication? *etc.*).

Finally, psychoanalytic diagnosis includes additional issues: structural organization of the personality, character types, Ego functions, unconscious phantasies, conflicts and defences, infantile relationships repeated in transference, vital situation and family dynamics, semiotics of the body, predominant fixated drives, psychosomatic functioning, *etc.*

Opposite to what happens in the theoretical framework of medicine, psychoanalysts tend to consider the skin and the psyche as if they were inseparable. Consequently, they apply concepts like "Ego – skin" [8] or "Psychic skin" or "defensive skin" when they do analytic work with people suffering from personality disorders and psychoses but not necessarily from a skin disorder. For example, Schmidt names 'thin-skinned' and 'thick-skinned' the narcissism of some schizophrenic patients with extreme 'defences of the Self' [26].

As we mentioned above, E Bick called "second skin" a substitute for the failed skin container function.

Gupta and Gupta showed how many overlaps and difficulties exist to frame the syndromes clearly delimited in dermatology with the parameters, boundaries and diagnoses thought by psychiatrists for mental disorders [27].

The analyst's experience is very similar: on one hand, he must not forget the parameters of medicine and psychiatry to evaluate the patient before deciding the beginning of a psychoanalytic therapy. On the other hand, his lens - and more than his lens, his listening – allows him to define concepts, parameters and types of patients whose subjective richness cannot be found in the generalization of the Diagnostic and Statistic Manual of Mental Disorders.

Additionally, although it is important to distinguish between primary psychiatric disorders and multifactorial skin diseases. In all cases a true psychosomatic approach means to prevent the patient to become fixated on a purely somatic/physical understanding of illness [28]. This prevention must be done not only with dermatitis artefacta or body dysmorphic disorder (which belong to the group of primary psychiatric disorders) but also with Psoriasis, Atopic Dermatitis, alopecia areata, acné, *etc.* (which belong to the group of multifactorial kin diseases).

Anzieu has a very precise clinical objective when he proposes that psychoanalysis in cases of difficult pathologies - narcissistic neurosis or a borderline cases -, should allow us to assess which Ego function is the missing one and to see what kind of analytic work can be done in order to fill the lack and to re-establish the missing function of the Ego. The author underlines a difference between working with the psychic contents (as with neurotic patients) and working with the psychic container (as with borderline patients). In the latter case the job is to repair the failures and to re-establish the function of the container.

A great contribution has been made by Hart, Gieler, Kusnir and Tausk when they say that “the diagnosis of the underlying psychiatric conditions in psychodermatology involves several dimensions. Evaluating each of these provides the psychodermatologist with more opportunities to develop an effective treatment” [28].

Some of the dimensions they described are: The level of functioning, the different physical and psychosocial stressors influencing the level of functioning, the concurrent affective components and the secondary gain.

The levels of functioning are based on a psychoanalyst´s work: Otto Kernberg [25]. He proposes the existence of three comprehensive structural organizations: the neurotic organization, the borderline organization and the psychotic organization of the personality. These organizations mediate between the etiologic factors and the direct behavioral manifestations of the disease and are reflected in the predominant characteristics of the patient, mainly regarding:

- His level of identity integration.
- The kinds of defensive operations usually employed.
- His capacity for the reality test.

These characteristics can be observed in the Table **1** (*Adapted from Kernberg and Garza Guerrero with modifications)* [25, 29].

Table 1. Mean PDI values of the field test after treatment with tobacco preparation.

	Identity	Defensive organization	Reality test
Neurotic organization of the personality	Integrated. Stable object relationships. Representations of himself and the objects accurately delimited	Repression. High level of defences based in the repression.	Conserved +++
Borderline organization of the personality	Poorly integrated. Unstable object relationships Diffusion of the identity.	Splitting. Disavowal. Primitive Defences.	Conserved +
Psychotic organization of the personality	Not integrated. Undifferentiated relationships.	Splitting. Disavowal. Repudiation. Primitives Defences.	Seriously altered. Confusional

These structural criteria can complement ordinary descriptions of the patients either behavioural or phenomenological [25] and contribute to the differential diagnosis.

The proposed comprehensive structural organizations do not imply a reductionism: for example, "to say that a patient is a borderline only connotes that from the point of view of structural development and analysis, his performance reflects certain defects in the integration and differentiation of intra psychic structures, characterizing a borderline level of personality organization. The style or pattern, however, may be narcissistic, childish, paranoid, schizoid, sadomasochistic, cyclothymic, *etc.*" [29]. The type of transference in the analysis with the therapist is an additional important feature for the diagnosis.

If the general dermatologist (*i.e.* not the psychodermatologist) is able to differentiate the neurotic, borderline and psychotic levels of functioning, this will be of much help to manage the consultation having a "macroscopic" psychiatric/psychological viewpoint, while at the same time keeping his usual dermatology "lens". And what about the analyst? Once he counts with the dermatologic diagnosis given by the dermatologist, plus the psychiatric diagnosis and the assessment of the personality organization established by him during the interview, the analyst enters another level of analysis, typifying the kind of unconscious conflicts, wishes and emotions that the patient expresses through his/her complaints and symptoms and detecting the defence mechanisms that the patient uses to cope with reality, with stress and with his disease. If an interdisciplinary team is working, as every prescription has an unconscious meaning, the team can help the dermatologist to choose the treatment when many possibilities are available and can give him skills to improve the doctor-patient relationship [10].

4. Skin Symptoms and Pathologies

To begin to understand skin patients we must accept that abandonment is experienced as a wound. A wound threatening to reopen again, possibly more than once and thus making the patient feel in danger, exposed to the risk of being abandoned or attacked at any time. Attachment and rejection, love and hatred, can therefore coexist [30].

Psychoanalytic works like that of Sylvie Consoli have shed light on how these experiences are pathologically processed by the patient determining the necessity to build a sort of protective barrier that ultimately affects his skin.

Another important issue is to be aware of the link between the skin, the consciousness and the memories. Instead of building an image of the other in his memory, the patient tries to carry a feature of the other on the skin, much like individuals who get tattooed or fans who once they could touch their idol, try to avoid washing their hands ever again. Carrying the other on the skin or soaking up his image, creates the illusion of a symbiotic fusion [31].

Hence, family relationships, mourning, attachment style, must be considered as variables that intervene in the disease evolution as well as inflammation mediators do. Life events could be chained in a sort of cascade as well as cytokines, skin cells, lymphocytes and neuropeptides are chained in inflammation processes.

a. Itching

According to M Schur "itching may be experienced as a concomitant or an equivalent of a variety of affects. In the analysis of itching he emphasises its compulsive character, the masturbatory basis, the feelings of guilt and self-punishment and the mechanisms of punishing someone else by means of self-destruction". "The gratification produced by scratching exceeds the mere elimination of displeasure caused by itching, and in some cases, it even comes to be the only or the main way of sexual gratification" [32].

Pichon Riviere considered the skin as an erotogenic zone and the scratching as an action in search of erotogenic satisfaction. Itching has been considered for him to be a form of masturbation with an intense repression of genital life [4].

We can find in Freud's Works a lot of references on itching. He said that a sensation of itching or stimulation which is centrally conditioned is projected on to a peripheral erotogenic zone [9]. Analyzing "the rat man" he related the anal erotism with the irritation due to worms and the anal pruritus [33].

Ulnik states that there may be nothing more "itch-provoking" than loving or needing somebody one hates, or the reverse, hating oneself because one loves and needs someone who is "impossible" [34]. Thus, not only pleasure but also rage could be expressed and carried out by itching and scratching.

b. Appendixes of the Skin

The wishes to incorporate the other or to merge him/her with parts of the Self can be manifested in attitudes aimed at the appendixes of the skin, such as the hair and the nails. Schur refers to a case in which he could appreciate, *in statu nascendi,* the development of trichotillomania in a one-year old child who had replaced the dummy for the pleasure of having hairs of his mother inside his mouth. This was later replaced by the action of pulling and sucking his own hair.

F Widder published a case report of alopecia areata in a child who slept in bed with their parents until the birth of her sister. When that happened, the parents decided to develop separation from his son in stages: first days he slept in a crib within the parents' room. Then, they took the crib to the child´s room but tied with a rope one leg of the crib to one leg of the parents' bed saying to their son to pull the rope to call them if he suffered from anxiety or woke at night. Finally, when her sister grew enough to be out of the parents´ room, they cut the rope that tied their bed with the boy´s crib. Since then, he has developed alopecia areata, as if his hair was the equivalent of the missing rope that bound his parents with him. The disease appears as a sign of the difficulty to bear the separation process among all this family members [35].

According to psychoanalytical theory, each separation or lost out of the body could be experienced as a sort of "castration", that means the loss of something very important of the body or the self. So, it has been said that the illusion of some alopecia areata and universal alopecia patients that the hair will grow again transmits a fantasy of avoiding the consequences of castration, because what has been cut or has fallen can re-appear in the same way as it was before [36].

M. Delplanque says that the alopecias appear as the senseless symptoms of the anxiety of another person whose symbiotic proximity is looked for by the patient. The patient, unconscious of it, was compelled to remain captive within the other´s enjoyment" [37].

JM López Sanchez, applying Roscharch test, psycho-drama technique, and psycho dynamically oriented interviews has described inhibition of aggression and behaviours of submission and passivity as personality traits of alopecia areata patients [38].

c. Self Inflected Lesions

Koblenzer has linked self infliction of lesions with borderline personality structures and with the inability to develop mature relationships.

"They use their lesions to obtain the attention and the nurturing they desperately need to maintain contact with others, and thus to fill their emotional emptiness [22].

She says that other possible purposes of self-inflicted lesions maybe achieving a punishment for unconscious feelings of guilt, or giving way to displaced infantile rage.

P. Brun-Ney mentions two cases of self-inflicted lesions. In the first case, a teenager expresses with her cuts both her aggression against her mother, who is not the mother who was supposed to be and her displeasure against herself and her guilt. In the second case, the cuts on the skin are interpreted as a way of searching the continent function of the mother. In both cases, the self-inflicting behaviour is thought as a defensive move against either the psychotic regression, or the incestuous advance [39].

According to Consoli, the sacrifice by means of body injuries protects the subject from the other who is seen as the one who could cross the boundaries and thus penetrate the patient´s thoughts and privacy. As a symbol representing identity, the lost body reconquers itself through sacrifice and pain.

On the contrary, the secret of the self-injuring behavior, kept at all costs, jealously guarded, is no stolen by anyone, in order not to repeat the story from childhood: a story without privacy, without respect, without ownership over one's body and without consent over one´s own feelings. The skin lesions are, finally, a barrier, a protection, a paradoxical guarantee of integrity. Thanks to their being secretive, patients are separated and protected from us [40].

The task of an analyst is to find which emotions, fantasies, impressions and stories reenact the patient's current problem whether the latter consists of an overvalued idea, an obsession or a symptomatic action. The same task also encompasses understanding this re-enactment as an anagram that dot by dot, held by invisible lines, reproduces, in a deformed way, a body of childhood which has been abused, traumatized, unregistered, overwhelmed with excitement, or eroticized in a unique way [41].

There is one study carried out in Finland with a sample of 41 patients with prurigo nodularis interviewed by the same analyst [42]. He found childhood environments and early developmental years as harsh and emotionally restricted. Nearly all patients′ interviews had recollections of painful experiences filled with loneliness and a longing for warm contact with another human being.

d. Psoriasis

For Schur, it does not seem to be a fantasy to assume that, "...in certain constellations in which a profound regression of the Ego is produced, the skin works as a transmitter of primitive symbols of thought, discourse and action. In these regressive states, the differentiation between the Self and the object can be vague, regression can be very deep, narcissistic and exhibitionistic tendencies can prevail, and the skin can be treated as a part of the Self and, simultaneously, as part of the external object. In three cases of psoriasis treated by him, he claims to have found in the patients a great confusion regarding their own identity, a product of ambivalent identifications with the parents. Once the lesion has established itself, its morphologic characteristics, its localisation and the secondary assessment that can be produced about it can influence or add elements to the identity confusion" [3]. "Once the symptom has established itself, it acts as a focal point of convergence for different pathological mechanisms" [3]. Following Schur, Ulnik summarizes that every somatic disease attracts narcissistic libido and any response to an organic disease shall involve a temporal or permanent regression that affects all the psychic structures. Whichever the cause that precipitates the dermatological disorder might be, the result will not depend only on the seriousness of the organic disease, but on the level of mental health at the time when the disease started and also during its evolution [34].

J Ulnik *et al.* have studied psoriasis patients with the "affective distances test", developed to assess the quality of bondings - in terms of distance - between the patient and the others. They have found unconscious fears of fusion and indiscrimination.

Regarding doctor – patient relationship they have found that the patient's need to feel loved, protected, or attached to others, influences the type of bond they have with their doctor. Thus, they confuse physical proximity and medical care: being clingy or getting the doctor always present means being in the doctor´s mind and therefore better treated. They also could equate the doctor´s office as if it were their home and expect the doctor to be as a family member or friend. Otherwise, they can develop a defence against the fusion with an attitude of detachment and avoidance that results from an unconscious fear of invasion. Sometimes, an alternation between both attitudes – on one hand an excessive demand with a symbiotic style and on the other hand detachment and avoidance – is observed, producing confusion in the medical team [47].

In his book Theatres of the body, J Mc Dougall described patients with somatic diseases having the fantasy that there is only one sex or one body for two and the primitive fear of the loss of body boundaries, sense of personal integrity or sexual identity [6].

Regarding the sexual relationship in psoriasis patients, several authors say that their involvement in sexuality does not depend on the degree of severity of symptoms [44] and could even be unrelated to the genital location [45]. According to them, concerns about the texture and appearance of other non-genital skin sites play an important role in sexuality [46]. In addition, the sense of intimacy, strongly related with the whole skin, is a clue in this issue.

Magin *et al.* [46] studied the speech of patients through semi-structured interviews and report cases in which sexual concern is associated with the fear that the partenaire crosses their barriers or the phantasy of being exposed. They mention a case who conceived the sexuality as "something magnetic".

With the affective distances test, we found that patients´ fears of losing the integrity, getting inside the other or making him or her disappear usually generate an avoidant distance when facing sexual contact. This can occur in two ways: a) Fear of disappearing within the other: "A sexual contact has to be gluing, consuming, absorbing until disappearing"; b) Fear to make the other disappear or to overwhelm the other: "If a person attracts me, I try to approach, but try not to be heavy and not to be too over her" [47].

Finally, we could propose the hypothesis that sexual difficulties in these patients are not only consequences or "sequelae" of psoriasis but manifestations of deeper alterations related to the Ego-body, the identity and the function of the skin as a boundary, a container, a barrier of protection and a screen that shows who each other is [47].

e. Vitiligo

Regarding vitiligo patients Stelio de Carvalho Neto (2011) wonders: Can vitiligo be analogous to the product of the “aggressive” creation of an artist? Vitiligo is a self-injury involving the destruction of melanocytes. What if aggression were comparable to the aggression of the sculptor's chisel on a block of marble? What if that aggression engenders a contour instead of annihilating a contour already established [48]?

Quoting a verse from J L Borges - the Argentine writer - Carvalho makes an analogy: an already old and blind Borges touches his own face and explores it while he is in front of a mirror which returns an invisible image. In the same way Carvalho states that psychosomatic skin lesions could also be the effect of blindness in the mirror – a mirror function needed to build and own the body image.

Then, he states his strongest hypothesis: vitiligo could “make” a body in a bodiless person, and he proposes that there could be two types of vitiligo: vitiligo-with- a body and vitiligo- without- a body [48]. The first ones are patients that can symbolize their problems and express their feelings through their symptoms as conversion disorder patients usually do, and the second ones are more primitive patients – in psychological terms – who build their body image creating - through their lessions - a body that was previously absent. Opposite to what it seems, in his opinion vitiligo doesn´t “delete”, but “draws”.

What about patients who develop vitiligo and then tattoo themselves to cover their spots? Does it mean that vitiligo first engenders a body so that later the patient can tattoo that body? [48]. Seeing the Canadian model Winnie Harlow and the announcements about her: "Canadian Winnie Harlow is one of the most important models in the country and is projected as a great figure in the world of fashion" we can figure out the way that vitiligo "makes" a body.

My opinion is that although vitiligo perhaps makes a body, at the same time shows a need to remove something else. In this sense we agree with Carvalho Neto when referring to the lack of anxiety and spontaneous demand in vitiligo patients sent to psychotherapy he says: Some people do not need to look at their own body to thread the image of their suffering. But there are others who scrutinize their meat with their looking to find a picture of their anxiety. If vitíligo has already warranted a *"mise en scène"*, why announcing the anxiety? [48]. Carvalho's idea of diseases with a body and diseases without a body leads us to inquire: on what basis is the disease installed? Which is the body that is being attacked or healed? Which functions or body parts are invaded, not represented, not completely built yet, "deleted", *etc.*

f. Allergy

Symbiosis and Identity:

According to Noemí L. de Canteros, the hyper-sensitive reaction of the immune system is a defence reaction, an exaggerated one, of an identity that could not reach an adequate individuation [49].

The identity that feels threatened is a syncretic or symbiotic kind of identity, based on "we", and the hyper-sensitive reaction might be the way of expressing a wish and the fear to the situation that requires a change in this identity and a passage from the symbiotic state to individual identity [49].

In allergic patients, differentiating the relationship with the other from identification can become really difficult, and the biological model of the relationships they hold can be that of the host-parasite relationship [49].

As these patients are trapped in their development by an extreme dependence, they reject independent life. They have the tendency to delegate to their symbiotic *partenaires* the tasks of adaptation, defence and competition, and therefore, they remain away from the changes in the world around them and have particular difficulties in facing new situations. The prototype could be a fearful person, who avoids any situation that implies responsibility, a person who always expects to be in familiar grounds, and when a situation of change arises, he reacts in a hyper-sensitive way [49].

This author has great experience working with asthmatic patients, but she also mentions atopic patients in general, and it is well known the alternation between asthma and eczema that some of the patients with these characteristics show.

Object Relationship

In "the allergic object relation", Marty develops some ideas which often agree with those of Canteros, which are of a later date. According to Marty, the allergic patient´s primordial wish is to get as near as possible to the object until he is confused with it. To be able to achieve this, he takes two actions: first, the attraction of the object, and second, the conditioning of it.

The attraction of the object involves a confusion of the subject with the object since the subject has own difficulties in establishing his/her own boundaries. In an example, Marty mentions a woman who used to say that she loved being caressed and that was why she loved cats. When Marty pointed out to her that in fact what she liked was to caress, because cats do not caress, and she herself was the one carrying out the action, she replied: "Yes, but cats rub against ourselves and caress us when we caress them".

When there is confusion in a common unity between the subject and the object, the former becomes unable to conceive a distance adequately, and this confusion causes massive projection or confusion of the subject with his environment.

Conditioning is a progressive inter-penetration that occurs throughout time. He mentions a patient with eczema who used to say: "What I want is that the boundaries with the others disappear, perhaps that is why I'm looking for physical contact. If I touch someone else's skin, I become mixed up with him…" [50]. This is about making boundaries disappear by means of projection and identification.

According to Marty, relationships can be established at different levels; such as sensory, motor, fantasmatic, intellectual, *etc.* The allergic reaction could be the manifestation of establishing a relationship at the humoral level.

The disease can appear when unleashing regressive mechanisms that activate this humoral level. This is what happens when facing two typical circumstances: first, when an invested object reveals a characteristic of his own with which the allergic subject cannot identify. Second, when two equally invested objects manifest incompatibilities with each other. Consequently, the subject feels torn and incompatible with himself; since he has become fused with both objects at the same time and these do not get on together.

Regression can be interrupted when the allergy irrupts. If this does occur, episodes of depersonalisation can be triggered.

The relationship with the doctor or with the analyst can also interrupt regression and can even prevent the allergy from arising. The problem is that any proof of independence or new qualities in the doctor can even go beyond the patient´s adaptability [50].

Perhaps if we take Marty's claims as a starting point, we are able to explain the usual hyper-sensitivity of some patients who, due to either any disagreeable detail, no matter how unimportant it might be, or to any small disagreement with the analyst, are capable of giving up treatment, thus spoiling the achievements reached so far.

Psychosis and Spaces of Reciprocal Inclusions

Similar to Canteros and Marty, and agreeing with many theoretical coincidences, Mahmoud Sami-Ali refers to the skin mainly when he talks about allergy. According to Sami-Ali [51] the world of allergy is built in such a way that the body and the world form an equivocal mass, where "every relationship is the contact of a skin that touches another skin and where the active and the passive, to touch and being touched are considered to be equivalent".

In order to introduce a boundary, a difference, a polarity, it is needed to create a distance exactly where it is difficult to do it. That can only occur if the allergic relationship with the world is displaced regarding the tactile sense giving place to a distancing created by the visual and the auditory senses.

Every allergy could be a questioning of what oneself is and what oneself is not [51]. Personal identity in its most profound aspect, at the origins of subjectivity can be at stake. The "bet" of the allergic patient would be to reduce everything to the identical, and his crisis could erupt when the other reveals himself in his otherness through "tearing himself off".

Until here Sami-Ali´s theory does not seem to be too different from that of Marty´s. Perhaps his contribution to this subject is the relationship he makes between allergy and psychosis, proposing that when the allergic patient is faced with a contradiction, because of the failure of the unique and identical to himself relationship that he is seeking, a no way out situation that sets the start of a psychotic elaboration might be generated [51].

Psychosis could attack the root of the contradiction itself, turning the contradictory into the identical and resulting in the characteristic space of delirium, where the notion of "inside" is considered equal to the notion of "outside" and the part, equal to the whole. Sami-Ali called "spaces of reciprocal inclusions" [52] to these kinds of spaces in which the duplication of the same within the self is produced, as it usually occurs when a TV presenter speaks with a monitor behind him in which he himself is speaking with a monitor behind him, and so forth [53].

Sami-Ali proposes a dialectic of substitution of psychosis and somatic disease which happens to be extremely useful for clinical work with skin patients with borderline or psychotic organization of the personality.

5. Therapy

Consoli's advice is as follows: before treating patients´ emotions – their oedipal emotions – sufficiently sound and reliable limits have to be established in order to contain them [40].

The couch promotes words exchange and interrupts other usual channels of exchange and communication. Nevertheless, due to the anxieties and regression this method generates, psychoanalysis using the couch should be indicated only after assessing the patient's ability to tolerate such frustration and only once the relationship has become significant and stable enough. In the meantime, psychoanalysis could also be developed face to face, as Freud said: "to alloy the pure gold of analysis freely with the copper of direct suggestion" [54].

a. Present Conflicts and Patient's Motivation

Relationship between psyche and soma is very complex. Therefore, proposing that one kind of psychotherapy outstands the rest or indicating a unique approach for each disease turns out to be a simplification that leaves aside the fact that we don´t treat diseases but sick people.

In the same way as a complex cascade of pro-inflammatory events take place in a psoriasis plaque, a complex cascade of psychopathologic factors intervene in a psychosomatic chain. In the same way as biologic agents act at different levels stopping inflammation , different psychotherapies act at different levels modifying either coping strategies, psychological consequences of the disease, psychological or psychosocial trigger factors, psychodynamics (defence mechanisms, unconscious patterns, transference – counter transference processes, *etc.*).

Psychoanalysis states that our Ego is like a servant of three severe masters: the external world (reality), the inner world, which is unconscious and pushes for drives of satisfaction and the Superego that represents our moral rules, our parents and educators teachings and wishes, and our ideals. Our symptoms have unconscious meanings and are related to our childhood and sexuality. The doctor-patient relationship repeats unconscious models taken from our family relationships and upbringing time.

Thus, one of the first tasks to do is taking a psychosomatically oriented history. In psychoanalytic terms, it means some face-to-face, semi-directed interviews in order to define the consultation motive and to gather the details of the vital history of the patient and of his disease. Eliciting the patient's beliefs and explanations of his or her disease, and encouraging him to express his subjective and emotional experience related to the disease, we obtain valuable data beyond the disease. That means that unconscious memories, infantile traumas, repressed ideas, supressed feelings, childish bonds, *etc.* are usually projected on the body, the disease and the doctor – patient relationship.

The ideal, - tough very difficult to fulfil – is the shared consultation. Ulnik *et al.* have implemented in a psoriasis centre a method which includes the presence of a dermatologist and a psychoanalyst in the same office [34]. Some groups in other hospitals and institutions are doing the same (H Ramirez in Sao Paulo Brazil at Instituto da Pele [43], E. Rottenberg in Buenos Aires, at Children´s Hospital Gutierrez, *etc.*).

When telling the doctor about the history of his illness, when taking off his clothes, when paying the fee, the patient makes comments and has patterns of behaviour which the dermatologist 'rules out´, but the psychoanalyst can understand and take advantage of in the subsequent treatment.

In general, the patient does not remain silent while the dermatologist examines him. He usually makes comments about his body, his lesions and also his 'defects', which are exposed with his nakedness. The same occurs with the prescription of a treatment: patients who show resistance to it usually make comments about its side effects, its physical characteristics (odour, colour, consistency), its cost or its lack of effectiveness.

Within all these comments, we can find fantasies (sometimes conscious and others unconscious) which manifest themselves; they interact with the disease, determining the patterns of behaviour and irrational attitudes that make each case unique and which are of incredible value in psychotherapy.

What the psychoanalyst hears in the doctor's consulting room gives him the possibility to infer that there are unconscious factors which play a role in:

- The motive and time of consultation.
- The self-destructive patterns of behaviour that worsen the disease.
- The kind of complaint or suffering privileged by the patient.
- The acceptance or rejection of a treatment or a medicine.
- The location of the lesions.

Once the doctor collected sufficient information, a new difficult task begins: to motivate the patient to start a psychodynamic psychotherapy.

This happens not only with the analyst´s work but also with the dermatologist´s help and participation.

This help doesn´t mean the dermatologist has to "get rid of the patient", because things go better when the patient continues being a skin patient who has a place in the mind and the office of his dermatologist. Fortunately, the interdisciplinary work provides some tools and new points of view to the dermatologist.

Patients should not be confronted too early with the need of psychiatric or psychotherapeutic approaches. First, the dermatologist should create a stable, trusting relationship between him/her and the patient and explore the patient´s motivation to undergo psychotherapy.

There is a difficult "ride" from the physical symptoms or complaints to the psychosocial situation. It´s recommendable to increase the frequency of consultation visits. They can be used to know the history of the patient´s psychosocial situation – as extended as possible - , showing interest in it.

Patients usually expect a prescription for each consultation. But they tolerate not having one, if the dermatologist inverts the pattern: for example, when asking them to undergo lab tests before prescribing. The doctor can add a complaint diary as an indication and the one to fulfil the demand will be the patient, not him. Taking a simple QoL questionnaire (for example the DLQI) and showing the numeric result to the patient as it would be done with a blood analysis, helps the doctor to show with a concrete and numeric result the additional help that the patient needs.

Psychological healing is a process, not a surgery intervention. So, for a time, both dermatologist and psychoanalyst should tolerate not healing.

Patient's complaints are a part of his/her speech. They don´t imply the dermatologist's failure or that something is wrong. He shouldn´t take the complaints personally, Offering more and more useless prescriptions or unnecessary studies is a failed response. After that recognition, a support along the difficult path to healing is needed and the professional container function, patience, knowledge and comprehension are the tools to do that.

Some patients need to idealize their doctor. This should be accepted, but only if the doctor feels capable of bearing the fall that will happen sooner or later. The higher the idealization is, the more important the fall will be.

Even in patients with real somatic diseases, becoming fixated on a purely somatic/physical understanding of illness must be prevented.

Suggestion works better when it is used smartly: if canceling the symptoms or pathologic behavior is suggested directly, it will probably fail. Symptoms and disease are powerfully and strongly entangled like a fishing hook caught on a rock. Sometimes, cutting the line, forgetting the hook and using another bait is needed.

b. A Different Way of Psychoeducation

One way to obtain patient´s motivation is showing the relationship between the disease or the symptom and the present or past conflicts. But to be trustable, it is necessary not to explain but to play with the analogical parallelism. For example, if the patient is phobic and doesn't leave his home and at the same time suffers from alopecia areata, doctor can compare the person's behaviour with the hair "behaviour": both, hair and himself don't dear to come outside, to face the external world. If the patient is hippomaniac and suffers from psoriasis, it is useful to compare the acceleration of his speech and thinking and the acceleration of keratinocytes´ growing. All of this can be explained to the patient who will be very interested in learning about his cells´ "behaviour" or the underlying mechanisms of his disease. This enhances patient´s motivation to connect his attitudes with his disease although this connection is only metaphorical or artificially created by the psychotherapist and it´s not neither the cause nor the "meaning" or the explanation of the disorder.

c. Emotional Expression

Sometimes, patients have rage, resentment, aggression, hostility, *etc.*, emotions that are repressed or not expressed openly. Psychotherapy has the aim to facilitate them to express their feelings or to make them clear in the psychotherapeutic setting working them out both through the interaction and by interpretation.

There is not only a learned behavior pattern but also a conflict model underlying the symptom, which can be worked out with the patient. "Working out the unconscious elements by reflecting the transferences enables the patient to find a way to explain his or her disorder instead of simply working on the learned symptom reactions" [28].

The work with projection is usually very useful. It consists in detecting and describing the physical and emotional state of significant others around the patient, such as objects, pets, movie-characters and even friends and relatives. Once detected and described, these emotions have already been named. Therefore, linking them with the patient's life events will be easier.

The psychotherapist – as well as the dermatologist - must get to be recognized by the patient as someone else with whom to establish a relationship without danger of being invaded or disappearing after a separation. Simultaneously, the patient should find that his feelings and his self are validated and accepted

d. Objectives Specifically Designed for Skin Patients

Avoiding the Gaze Channel in Communication

Examining the patient, you think you are the one who looks, but at the same time you are looked at and evaluated. That´s the reason why the "wandering patients" or " Doctor – shopping" patients usually tell each new doctor - with detailed and acute observations - the failures and disappointing experiences with the previous others.

It is necessary to open a new communication channel. So, the first words must be: - "*Please, tell me what´s going on*" instead of : -"*Show me what´s going on*".

Separating the time of dialogue from the time of physical examination seems to be a good advice. Skin lesions are usually examined in detail, with a dermoscopy or a magnifier. Patient as a whole shouldn´t be observed in that way. Paradoxically, although the psychoanalytic technique suggests going to the couch, as we have already mentioned above [40] at the beginning psychoanalysis also could be developed face to face, to avoid the anxieties and regression this classical method might generate.

Modifying the Attachment Style

Who is the "real" patient? In many agglutinated families and with symbiotic partners it is difficult to find the answer to this question. Once the patient starts his analysis, he could probably repeat his attachment style with the analyst. The analysis of transference and counter transference is the best field to work this through, and it is very common to see that when the patient gains autonomy and develops his own criteria or goes after his realization wishes, another family member appears with a new disease… that could even be on the skin!

Stopping the Self-injuring Behaviour

Psychoanalysts are not used to giving behavioral indications or "homework", but use the setting and the transference-counter transference as a field where interpretations and some therapeutic actions can be done. Therefore, every self-injuring behavior which occurs during sessions should be incorporated and interpreted as part of the emotional world of the patient and as an indicator of what is happening with him at that moment. Considering this behavior as part of a non-verbal "language", it could be interpreted. On the other hand, establishing its interruption during the session could be licit too, to the extent that other communication modes are stimulated.

Re-building the Body Image

Firstly, iti s important to open many channels of communication so that the gaze is not the only channel or the most privileged one. Look at your patient, but not in the same way as he usually is being looked at. This means that building another image through your gaze can really help the patient a lot. If the patient insists in a "showing behavior" during psychotherapy as if the psychoanalyst were the same as a dermatologist – or even if a psychodermatologist who is also a dermatologist is in charge of the analysis – ask the patient to talk. Without under valuating his skin suffering, respond to the "show" as if the images of the skin were not enough to be understood.

There are patients who need to be seriously ill in order to feel they do have a body. They have built a characterological and affective shell as a defence mechanism in order not to feel hurt. In consequence, the symptoms of skin disease are a means of expression and awareness of their own emotional status. For example, a lesion characterized by its impenetrability and scabby surface might well soothe a patient who feels he has no body boundaries, and it could also provide him with the category of a "protective barrier".

Another strategy is using different dermatological treatments beyond their specific action, as concrete elements that can help the patient define the boundaries of his body, or provide self-representation and the categories of open-close, hard-smooth, clean-dirty, and so on.

CONCLUSION

Psychoanalytic evaluation can contribute to the dermatologic practice at many different levels: a) establishing the level of psychological/psychiatric functioning during the consultation; b) typifying the kind of unconscious conflicts and emotions that the patient expresses through his/her complaints and symptoms; c) detecting the defence mechanisms that the patient uses to cope with reality, with stress and with his disease; d) choosing the treatment taking into account the unconscious preferences and meanings of the prescriptions; and e) giving skills to improve doctor-patient relationship.

From a psychoanalytical point of view, almost all dermatological disorders can be considered psychodermatological disorders, because psychoanalytical conception is not based on the existence of an organic aetiology, or on the real somatic condition of the disease. in all of them – either self inflicted or not, delusional or real, chronic or acute - a psychodynamic approach can be made and can turn out useful, depending more on the patient than on the disorder itself.

The work of psychotherapy aims at helping patients become aware of their own feelings and express them, rather than through their bodies, through the process of psychical work out and building at the same time significant relationships.

The psychoanalytic perspective makes a contribution to the dermatology practice since it provides diagnostic dimensions, unconscious dynamics, fruitful explanations and therapeutic strategies. All these can help the physician recognize structural psychological needs in their patients. These needs are expressed through complaints, symptoms, behaviour and even the disease itself brought by patients to the consultation. Being aware of the different levels of diagnoses and communication gives very good clues about how to proceed, opens the door to explore a number of therapeutic options, enhances the physician-patient relationship and facilitates referral to psychotherapy when needed. Psychoanalytic psychotherapy can help skin patients to face their disease and, in some cases, can help them improve or even heal, if it is accompanied by the appropriate skin treatment given by the dermatologist. When the disease has become a means of emotional expression; a surrogate form of identity; or a defence against the mental illness or psychological suffering the patient feels unable to face, psychoanalytic psychotherapy could be of most help [10]. This suffering, like psychic suffering, is minimised by all, and can only be understood by those who have experienced it, or at least, by those who have analysed it with a non exclusively visual curiosity. Only in this way we can understand, interpret, accompany and mitigate in some way the misery internally experienced by patients and displayed on their skin.

NOTES

[1]Transference in psychoanalysis is the process by which the patient repeats with the analyst models of relationship and emotions from infantile origin that remain unconscious. The transference reactivates these models and is one of the main fields of the analyst´s work.

CONFLICT OF INTEREST

The author confirms that author has no conflict of interest to declare for this publication.

ACKNOWLEDGEMENTS

Declared none.

REFERENCES

[1] Ulnik J. Skin in psychoanalysis. Karnac Review Winter 2007; 12.

[2] International Psychoanalytical Association. Available from: http://www.ipa.org.uk/en/Psychoanalytic_ Treatment/About_psychoanalysis.aspx#WhoIs 2014.

[3] Schur M. Comments on the metapsychology of somatization. Psychosom Study Child 1955; 10: 119-64.

[4] Pichón-Rivière E. Aspectos psicosomáticos de la dermatología La Psiquiatría: Una Nueva Problemática Nueva Visión. 2nd ed., Buenos aires: Spanish 1980.

[5] Korovsky E. Aportes para la comprensión de la psoriasis. 9th Symposium of CIMP. Spanish

[6] McDougall J. Theatres of the Body. London: Free Association Books 1989.

[7] Freud S. The ego and the id; The Standard Edition of the Complete Psychological Works of Sigmund Freud. New York: W.W. Norton & Company Inc 1923; pp. (19): 12-66.

[8] Anzieu D. The Skin Ego. Yale Univ Press 1989.

[9] Freud S. Three Essays on Sexuality. The Standard Edition of the Complete Psychological Works of Sigmund Freud. New York: W.W. Norton & Company Inc 1905; p. (7): 130.

[10] Ulnik JC. Psychological evaluation of the dermatology patient: a psychoanalyst's perspective. Clin Dermatol 2013; 31(1): 11-7. [http://dx.doi.org/10.1016/j.clindermatol.2011.11.002] [PMID: 23245969]

[11] Freud S. Studies on Hysteria. The Standard Edition of the Complete Psychological Works of Sigmund Freud . New York: W.W. Norton & Company Inc 1893; pp. (2): 1-323.

[12] Freud S. Fragment of an analysis of a case of hysteria. The Standard Edition of the Complete Psychological Works of Sigmund Freud. New York: W.W. Norton & Company Inc 1905; pp. (7): 7-122.

[13] Bick E. The experience of the skin in early object-relations. Int J Psychoanal 1968; 49(2): 484-6. [PMID: 5698219]

[14] Lemma A. Under de Skin A Psychoanalytic Study of Body Modification. London: Routledge 2010.

[15] Consoli S. La tendresse. French: Paris: Odile Jacob 2003.

[16] Koblenzer CS. Psychotherapy for intractable inflammatory dermatoses. J Am Acad Dermatol 1995; 32(4): 609-12. [http://dx.doi.org/10.1016/S0190-9622(05)80001-5] [PMID: 7896951]

[17] Koblenzer CS. Successful treatment of a chronic and disabling dermatosis by psychotherapy. A case report and discussion. J Am Acad Dermatol 1986; 15(2 Pt 2): 390-3. [http://dx.doi.org/10.1016/S0190-9622(86)70186-2] [PMID: 3734189]

[18] Poot F, Antoine E, Gravellier M, *et al.* A case-control study on family dysfunction in patients with alopecia areata, psoriasis and atopic dermatitis. Acta Derm Venereol 2011; 91(4): 415-21. [http://dx.doi.org/10.2340/00015555-1074] [PMID: 21336474]

[19] Pines D. Skin communication: early skin disorders and their effect on transference and

countertransference. Int J Psychoanal 1980; 61(3): 315-23.
[PMID: 7440071]

[20] Lee CS, Koo J. Psychopharmacologic therapies in dermatology: an update. Dermatol Clin 2005; 23(4): 735-44.
[http://dx.doi.org/10.1016/j.det.2005.05.015] [PMID: 16112451]

[21] Ulnik J, Czerlowski M, *et al.* Psychodynamic strategies for dermatologic patients. World Congress of Dermatology. Buenos Aires. 2007.

[22] Koblenzer CS. Psychosomatic concepts in dermatology. A dermatologist-psychoanalyst's viewpoint. Arch Dermatol 1983; 119(6): 501-12.
[http://dx.doi.org/10.1001/archderm.1983.01650300055017] [PMID: 6859891]

[23] Grossbart T, Sherman C. Skin deep, A Mind/Body Program for Healthy Skin. New Mexico: Health Press 1992; p. 140.

[24] Moss K. Contact at the borderline: psychoanalytic psychotherapy with EB patients. Br J Nurs 2008; 17(7): 449-55.
[http://dx.doi.org/10.12968/bjon.2008.17.7.29065] [PMID: 18642687]

[25] Kernberg O. Severe Personality Disorders: Psychotherapeutic Strategies. New Heaven, CT: Yale University Press 1993; p. 395.

[26] Schmidt M. Psychic skin: psychotic defences, borderline process and delusions. J Anal Psychol 2012; 57(1): 21-39.
[http://dx.doi.org/10.1111/j.1468-5922.2011.01949.x] [PMID: 22288539]

[27] Gupta MA, Gupta AK. Psychodermatology: an update. J Am Acad Dermatol 1996; 34(6): 1030-46.
[http://dx.doi.org/10.1016/S0190-9622(96)90284-4] [PMID: 8647969]

[28] Hart W, Gieler U, Kusnir D, *et al.* Clinical Management in Psychodermatology. Springer-Verlag: Berlin Heidelberg 2009.

[29] Garza Guerrero C. Problema de diagnostico diferencial en personalidades narcisistas: hacia un esquema de diagnostico integral. In: Revista de Psicoanálisis. Tomo XL 1983; pp. (5/6): 1093-23. Spanish

[30] Consoli SG. Dermatitis artefacta: a general review. Eur J Dermatol 1995; (5): 5-11.

[31] Ulnik J. Psychological aspects of the doctor-patient relationship in dermatology. Arch Arg Dermatol 1955; (1): 37-46. Spanish.

[32] Schur M. Comments on the metapsychology of somatization. Psychosom Study Child 1955; 10: 119-64.

[33] Freud S. Two Case Histories ('Little Hans' and the 'Rat Man'). The Standard Edition of the Complete Psychological Works of Sigmund Freud. New York: W.W. Norton & Company Inc. 1909; pp. (10): 153-251.

[34] Ulnik J. Skin in Psychoanalysis. London: Karnac Books 2007.

[35] Widder F. Expresiones orgánicas de conflicto y su relación con la histeria. Rev Psicoanal 1986; 43(5): 1067-82. [Spanish].

[36] Ulnik J, Chopitea de Fontan Balestra M. Alopecía areata: la ilusión de volver a crecer In: 11th IPSO Pre-congress. Buenos Aires 1991.

[37] Delplanque M. Des pelades dépasées. Psychologie Médicale, 1980; 12(2): 3936.

[38] López Sánchez JM. Exploración en psicodrama de pacientes alopécicos. Resúmenes de patología psicosomátical . Granada: Círculo de Estudios Psicopatologicos 1985.

[39] Brun-Ney P. Les conduites d'auto-destruction cutanée chez les adolescentes. Psychologie Médicale, 1980; 12(2): 345-7.

[40] Consoli SG. The case of a young woman with dermatitis artefacta: The course of the analysis. Derm Psychosom 2001; (2): 1-7.

[41] Nasio JD. Mi cuerpo y sus imágenes. Spanish: Buenos Aires: Paidós 2008.

[42] Valtola J. A psychiatric and psychodynamic investigation of LCO (Prurico Nodularis Hyde) patients. Acta Derm Venereol Suppl (Stockh) 1991; 156: 49-52.
[PMID: 2048377]

[43] Aragao e Ramirez H, Carvalho Assadi T, Lenz Dunker C. A pele como litoral Fenomeno psicossomático e psicanálise. Portuguese: Sao Paulo - Brasil: Annablume 2011.

[44] Sampogna F, Gisondi P, Tabolli S, Abeni D. Impairment of sexual life in patients with psoriasis. Dermatology (Basel) 2007; 214(2): 144-50.
[http://dx.doi.org/10.1159/000098574] [PMID: 17341864]

[45] Ludwig MWB, Oliveira MSO, Müller MC, Moraes JD. Qualidade de vida e localização da lesão em pacientes dermatológicos. Anais Brasileiros de Dermatologia 2009; 84(2): 143-50.
[http://dx.doi.org/10.1590/S0365-05962009000200007] [PMID: 19503982]

[46] Magin P, Heading G, Adams J, Pond D. Sex and the skin: a qualitative study of patients with acne, psoriasis and atopic eczema. Psychol Health Med 2010; 15(4): 454-62.
[http://dx.doi.org/10.1080/13548506.2010.484463] [PMID: 20677083]

[47] Ulnik J, Czerlowski MS, Meilerman DE, Murata C, Moure M, Salgado M, *et al.* Factores subjetivos en la sexualidad, el contacto y la calidad de vida de pacientes con psoriasis / Psoriatic patients: subjective factors in sexuality, contact, and quality of life. Anu. investig. - Fac. Psicol. Univ B Aires 2013; 20(2): 301-7.

[48] A pele como litoral. Fenomeno psicossomático e psicanálise. Portuguese: Sao Paulo - Brasil: Annablume 2011.

[49] Canteros N. Winnicott y la psicosomática. El Holding y el handling en la clínica con pacientes asmáticos y alérgicos. Buenos Aires: Encuentros: espacio Winnicott. 1997. Spanish

[50] Marty P. The allergic object relationship. Int J Psychoanal 1958; 39(2-4): 98-103.
[PMID: 13574943]

[51] Sami-Ali M. Pensar lo somático. Buenos Aires: Paidós: El imaginario y la patologia 1991. Spanish

[52] Sami-Ali M. Cuerpo real, cuerpo imaginario. Buenos Aires: Paidós: Para una epistemología psicoanalítica 1979. Spanish

[53] Ulnik J. Narcisismo y enfermedad somatica Actualidad psicológica 1993; 18(196): 18-21. Spanish

[54] Freud S. Lines of advance in psycho-analytic therapy In: The Standard Edition of the Complete Psychological Works of Sigmund Freud. New York: W.W. Norton & Company Inc 1993; 17: pp. 157-68.

CHAPTER 10

Building a Psychodermatology Clinic

Anna Zalewska-Janowska[1*], **Sol-Britt Lonne-Rahm**[2,3], **Sten Friberg**[4] and **Nordlind Klas**[3,5]

[1] *Psychodermatology Department, Medical University of Lodz, Poland*

[2] *Department of Dermatology, Mälarsjukhuset, Eskilstuna*

[3] *Dermatology and Venereology Unit, Department of Medicine, Solna, Karolinska Institutet, Stockholm*

[4] *Psykiatri Nordväst, Karolinska University Hospital, Solna*

[5] *Department of Dermatology, Karolinska University Hospital, Solna, Stockholm, Sweden*

Abstract: There is a need for a holistic view when treating dermatological patients. Dermatologists believe that psychiatric disorders are substantially less frequent than they actually are in many skin conditions. In many skin conditions the frequency of psychiatric disorders are underestimated by dermatologists. Diagnosing psychodermatological disorders, particularly depression, could in some cases, be lifesaving. In at least university teaching hospitals, psychodermatology clinics should function on a regular basis. The most natural location of such a clinic is within an ordinary dermatology clinic containing an interdisciplinary team of a dermatologist, psychiatrist, psychologist, social worker and experienced nurse. Instruments used include somatic examination, laboratory tests, and radiology facilities such as magnetic resonance, and neurophysiological examination. Treatment is composed of skin handling, emolliants, hydrocolloid dressings, ultraviolet light therapy, cognitive behavioural therapy, and/or pharmacotherapy using antidepressants or antipsycotics. These psychodermatological clinics, depending on refunding, may not be lucrative from the refunding perspective but they offer integrative patient care and may limit number of hospital admissions and improve the quality of life of these patients, this being the ultimate purpose.

* **Address correspondence by Anna Zalewska-Janowska:** Psychodermatology Department, Medical University of Lodz, 251 Pomorska, 92-213 Lodz, Poland; E-mail: Anna.Zalewska-Janowska@umed.lodz.pl

Klas Nordlind & Anna Zalewska-Janowska (Eds.)

Keywords: Anxiety, Clinic, Depression, Enquiries, Instruments, Laboratory tests, Outcome, Psychodermatology, Research.

BACKGROUND

The Need for a Psychodermatology Clinic

Dermatologists generally have a limited time for consultation by their patients, by tradition the flow of patients being high. In addition, the quality of the consultation from a holistic perspective may be limited, skin lesions being so visual. The skin disease may be worsened by psychological factors such as stress and depression and, on the other hand, the skin disease per se may lead to stress and depression due to influence on quality of life. It is important to identify which patients could receive more benefit from psychiatric intervention.

Dermatologists have a fairly good view about the impact of skin conditions on the quality of their patient′s life [1]. On the other hand, in many skin conditions the frequency of psychiatric disorders are underestimated by dermatologists [1, 2]. The prevalence estimates of psychiatric morbidity in dermatological outpatients range from 21 to 43% [2, 3].

Thus, anxiety, depression, body dysmorphic disorder (BDD) are often encountered. Depression in an outpatient dermatology setting has been estimated at having a prevalence of 34% and being comorbid with common skin disorders, including acne, atopic dermatitis, psoriasis, pruritus and urticaria [3]. In the study by Gee *et al.* [3] most physicians thought that they were capable to diagnose psychocutaneous disease, however, very few felt comfortable starting treatment with psychotropics or believed themselves being successful treating such conditions.

A substantial number of dermatologists are lacking training in psycho-dermatology, thus, many patients with psychocutaneous disorders are left untreated. Many patients are often resistant to psychiatric intervention and when they are adviced to see psychiatry, this often leads to termination of the treatment [3]. Thus, the major responsibility to recognize and treat psychiatric disorders is up to the treating dermatologist.

An added value to treating primary psychiatric disorders is the improvement of associated skin disorders. Accordingly psychiatric disorders due to skin disorders may also require treatment [4].

Assessing degree of stress, depression and anxiety using a simple 0-10 VAS scale before and during treatment can be a rough indicator of treatment progress. In addition, diagnosing the most common psychodermatological disorders, particularly depression, could in some cases, be lifesaving.

Psychodermatology Clinics

There are several examples of psychodermatology clinics [see, *e.g.*, 5 - 10]. Often the patients are seen by a combined team with a dermatologist/psychiatrist or psychologist. This is of particular importance since patients with primary psychodermatological disorders often do not want to have a psychiatric referral. The need for a psychodermatology multidisciplinary team for patients with dermatitis artefacta and artefactual skin disease from the initial consultation was pointed out by Mohandas *et al.* [6] at their regional psychodermatology clinic at the Royal London Hospital. With this early contract between the patient and both the dermatologist and psychiatrist, the clinical assessment could then be run over time.

In common for psychodermatology clinics is the difficulty to perform outcome based comparative studies.

A substantial number of patients default follow-up. Thus, most reports from these clinics in a retrospective way describe patients that have been admitted/treated by the clinics.

At the psychodermatology clinic in Singapore [5], the most common diagnosis among patients with primary psychiatric disorders was delusional infestation. 57.9% of the patients were compliant to the prescribed therapies, psychiatric medications or further psychiatric reviews. At the psychodermatology clinic in Manipal, India, the leading primary diagnosis was psoriasis, while the leading primary psychiatric disease was neurotic excoriations [7]. Thirty percent of the patients had stressors at the onset of their disease. At the Hadassah–Hebrew

University Medical Center at Ein, Israel, the patient meets with both a dermatologist and a clinical psychologist at the same time [9]. This clinic treats patients with cutaneous disorders such as psoriasis, atopic dermatitis, vitiligo, recurrent herpes, acne, lichen planus, trichotillomania, skin picking and delusional infestation. The psychodermatology clinic at Rehovot, Israel, is named ′a combined clinic` rather than a ′psychodermatology clinic`to obtain a neutral name (10). The need for time resource with 1-hour consultation, information, dermato-education and psycho-education is pointed out.

There are also, at several dermatological departments, eczema schools and life style receptions. These may be considered as early/naive psychodermatology platforms.

AIMS

Location of the Clinic

Which organization model of psychodermatology care should be the most effective? This item has been extensively dealt with by *e.g.* Aguilar-Duran *et al.* [8] based on their experience in UK.

In light of that the majority of these patients turn to common dermatology clinics, and in order not for the patients to become stigmatized, the natural location is within an ordinary dermatology clinic with a critical mass of patients and staff, most probably at a university hospital. It is important to educate and inform colleagues within such clinic and also referring private practitioner and family doctors about the clinic, being transparent. Residents should practice for a limited time period at the psychodermatology clinic. One should exclude "difficult" somatic patients from the clinic, and in which there is no added value by a referral to a psychodermatology clinic.

Staff

The staff should be interdisciplinary with a dermatologist interested in psychodermatology, psychiatrist, psychologist/psychotherapist, nurses, and social worker. Some of the patients should be seen at the same occasion by an interdisciplinary team. In this concept, it is important to remember that not all patients, especially those with delusional infestation or artefacts, want to be assessed by a team (at the same time). In such cases the patient should meet a separate doctor, dermatologist, as a front player/officer, who should offer the patient a meeting with interdisciplinary colleagues. Gentle handling by a nurse and social worker may have an important impact on patients with parasite delusions, being socially isolated. In stress-or depression-worsened inflammatory skin disease a team work should be the most efficient way to handle the patients. The interdisciplinary team may also have a beneficial/supportive role towards burn out syndrome within individuals of the same team.

Instruments

Of course of fundamental importance is to exclude infestations such as scabies and lice; this should be done at the first visit of the patient. In addition to a general somatic status (including central and peripheral nerve function), among laboratory tests, general blood samples (hemoglobin, white blood cells, platelets), liver enzymes, test for kidney function, thyroid hormones, test for fecal occult blood, screening for syphilis and HIV, are important, *e.g.*, in patients with delusional infestation, to exclude a somatic genesis. Moreover, important instruments are enquiries regarding degree of anxiety. State anxiety is measured by Hamilton Anxiety Rating Scale (HAM-A) and Hospital Anxiety and Depression Scale (HAD) [see ref. 11], depression using the Montgomery Åsberg Depression Rating Scale (MADRS)([12]), chronic stress/ exhaustion disorder, using Karolinska Exhaustion Disorder Scale)(KED) [13], also personality traits using such as Swedish Universities Scales of Personality (SSP) [14]. Magnetic resonance tomography (MR) is of value to be able to exclude brain processes/brain atrophy in patients with parasite delusions or general pruritus. In this respect also neurophysiological investigation might be of value to exclude neurological disease.

Patient Security

It is important to pay respect to legal aspects-local law and inform the patient-be empathetic and at the same time objective. Keep nomination neutral in order to destigmatize. Inform the patients about the clinic, but do not exaggerate, and keep distance. The doctors should be prepared for patient´s frustration and contact with legal authorities/patients organizations. In addition, a substantial number of patients default follow-up. Facing patients with a different cultural background demand a special taking care of, and in this context it may be important to involve staff with the same cultural/linguistic background as the patient.

Treatments

When meeting primarily a dermatologist, the patient, depending on the degree of suffering, may face different treatments, *e.g.*, local skin care by a trained nurse including titration of an optimal emollient, hydrocolloids as an artificial barrier, medical baths, UV treatment. UV treatment in this context also might have an antidepressive effect. Discussion with a social worker may be of particular value in patients with delusional infestation, in order to identify mechanisms such as social isolation. A trained nurse might be able to offer behavioural therapy, such as habit reversal, in order to decrease patients scratching. Antistress regimens, such as *via* cognitive behavioural therapy at individual or group level, through a psychologist/psychotherapist might be of value. Patients with stress worsening of their eczema may be able to structurize and find their stressors. For a minority of patients, dynamic psychotherapy might be of value. If no success with such treatments then psychopharmacological trials may be run using mixed monoamine uptake inhibitors, serotonin transporter inhibitors, or antipsychotics such as aripiprazol, risperidone, and haloperidol. Patients at a psychodermatology clinic may after a visit be handled by their local dermatologist/family doctor.

Research

Since a psychodermatology clinic probably often is located within university hospitals, it is natural that the activity should be tied to research, with possibilities to especially involve psychiatry, psychology, neurology, radiology, *etc.* Of course areas, such as stress and inflammation, are feasible in this respect due to the patient´s cognition/compliance, but also patients with delusional infestation should be of high interest, the patients being their own controls. Research may in the long run lead to individualized treatment for these patients.

Evaluation

Life quality enquires such as Dermatology Life Quality Index (DLQ1) enquiry [15] is important. In addition, anxiety and depression scales may be used. The number of skin lesions may be quantified. In patients with delusional infestation, the time that the patients spend per day thinking about the parasites may be a measure, as well as the quality of night sleep. However, we must be aware that a number of such patients probably will be frustrated due to their disease not being recognized as a somatic disease. Measuring outcomes will be a most necessary tool to motivate the existence of a psychodermatology clinic.

CONFLICT OF INTEREST

The authors confirm that they have no conflict of interest to declare for this publication.

ACKNOWLEDGEMENTS

Declared none.

REFERENCES

[1] Sampogna F, Picardi A, Melchi CF, Pasquini P, Abeni D. The impact of skin diseases on patients: comparing dermatologists' opinions with research data collected on their patients. Br J Dermatol 2003; 148(5): 989-95.
[http://dx.doi.org/10.1046/j.1365-2133.2003.05306.x] [PMID: 12786831]

[2] Picardi A, Abeni D, Mazzotti E, *et al.* Screening for psychiatric disorders in patients with skin diseases: a performance study of the 12-item General Health Questionnaire. J Psychosom Res 2004; 57(3): 219-23.
[http://dx.doi.org/10.1016/S0022-3999(03)00619-6] [PMID: 15507245]

[3] Gee SN, Zakhary L, Keuthen N, Kroshinsky D, Kimball AB. A survey assessment of the recognition and treatment of psychocutaneous disorders in the outpatient dermatology setting: how prepared are we? J Am Acad Dermatol 2013; 68(1): 47-52.
[http://dx.doi.org/10.1016/j.jaad.2012.04.007] [PMID: 22954748]

[4] Shenefelt PD. Psychodermatological disorders: recognition and treatment. Int J Dermatol 2011; 50(11): 1309-22.
[http://dx.doi.org/10.1111/j.1365-4632.2011.05096.x] [PMID: 22004480]

[5] Chung WL, Ng SS, Koh MJ, Peh LH, Liu T-T. A review of patients managed at a combined psychodermatology clinic: a Singapore experience. Singapore Med J 2012; 53(12): 789-93.
[PMID: 23268151]

[6] Mohandas P, Bewley A, Taylor R. Dermatitis artefacta and artefactual skin disease: the need for a psychodermatology multidisciplinary team to treat a difficult condition. Br J Dermatol 2013; 169(3): 600-6.
[http://dx.doi.org/10.1111/bjd.12416] [PMID: 23646995]

[7] Shenoi SD, Prabhu S, Nirmal B, Petrolwala S. Our experience in a psychodermatology liaison clinic at manipal, India. Indian J Dermatol 2013; 58(1): 53-5.
[http://dx.doi.org/10.4103/0019-5154.105310] [PMID: 23372214]

[8] Aguilar-Duran S, Ahmed A, Taylor R, Bewley A. How to set up a psychodermatology clinic. Clin Exp Dermatol 2014; 39(5): 577-82.
[http://dx.doi.org/10.1111/ced.12360] [PMID: 24934911]

[9] Elliman W. Mind over skin. Hadassah magazine Febr 2013. Available from: http://www.hadassahmagazine.org/2013/02/27/medicine-mind-skin/

[10] Orion E, Feldman B, Ronni W, Orit B-A. A psychodermatology clinic: the concept, the format, and our observations from Israel. Am J Clin Dermatol 2012; 13(2): 97-101.
[http://dx.doi.org/10.2165/11630950-000000000-00000] [PMID: 22251230]

[11] Stein DJ, Lopez AG. Effects of escitalopram on sleep problems in patients with major depression or generalized anxiety disorder. Adv Ther 2011; 28(11): 1021-37.
[http://dx.doi.org/10.1007/s12325-011-0071-8] [PMID: 22057726]

[12] Svanborg P, Åsberg M. A comparison between the Beck Depression Inventory (BDI) and the self-rating version of the Montgomery Asberg Depression Rating Scale (MADRS). J Affect Disord 2001; 64(2-3): 203-16.
[http://dx.doi.org/10.1016/S0165-0327(00)00242-1] [PMID: 11313087]

[13] Besèr A, Sorjonen K, Wahlberg K, Peterson U, Nygren A, Åsberg M. Construction and evaluation of a self rating scale for stress-induced exhaustion disorder, the Karolinska Exhaustion Disorder Scale. Scand J Psychol 2014; 55(1): 72-82.
[http://dx.doi.org/10.1111/sjop.12088] [PMID: 24236500]

[14] Gustavsson JP, Bergman H, Edman G, Ekselius L, von Knorring L, Linder J. Swedish universities Scales of Personality (SSP): construction, internal consistency and normative data. Acta Psychiatr Scand 2000; 102(3): 217-25.
[http://dx.doi.org/10.1034/j.1600-0447.2000.102003217.x] [PMID: 11008858]

[15] Finlay AY, Khan GK. Dermatology Life Quality Index (DLQI)--a simple practical measure for routine clinical use. Clin Exp Dermatol 1994; 19(3): 210-6.
[http://dx.doi.org/10.1111/j.1365-2230.1994.tb01167.x] [PMID: 8033378]

SUBJECT INDEX

D

K

L

M

N

O

P

S

T

www.ingramcontent.com/pod-product-compliance
Lightning Source LLC
Chambersburg PA
CBHW050825220326
41598CB00006B/310

* 9 7 8 1 6 8 1 0 8 3 0 2 5 *